Aromat[illegible]py Alchemy

Guide to Foundational Knowledge of All Things Essential Oils

By Sydney Brown

Aromatherapy Alchemy

GUIDE TO FOUNDATIONAL KNOWLEDGE OF ALL THINGS ESSENTIAL OILS

by Sydney Brown

Published by TLM Publishing House

5905 Atlanta Highway, Alpharetta GA.
https://www.ttpublishinghouse.com

Contents

Introduction:

Hey there! Welcome to the world of essential oils—a place where nature's aromatic wonders can enhance well-being in countless ways. Whether you're just starting out or already knee-deep in the essential oils business, this book is your shortcut to gaining a solid understanding and boosting your confidence.

We're here to help you cut through the confusion and save you months of trial and error. Our aim is to equip you with a foundational knowledge that'll not only enrich your own journey but also enable you to assist others more effectively.

So, let's kick things off by exploring the basics of essential oils, demystifying their extraction, and breaking down what makes a good-quality oil. No jargon, just plain talk to set you on the right path.

As we move along, we'll uncover the diverse benefits of these oils. Think physical wellness, emotional balance, and even a touch of spirituality. Plus, we'll delve into the intriguing history of essential oils, tracing their roots back to ancient times.

Safety first, right? We'll guide you through essential oil safety and usage, ensuring you and those you share them with are in good hands. And while we won't be spoon-feeding you recipes, we'll empower you with the know-how to create your blends based on your needs and preferences.

By the time you're done here, you'll have the confidence to navigate the world of essential oils like a pro. Whether you're just in it for personal passion or diving headfirst into business, this knowledge will be your compass.

So, let's get started on this practical journey. You're about to shave months off the learning curve and discover how these oils can truly enrich your life and the lives of those you connect with. Ready to dive in? Great! Let's roll.

The History of Essential Oils: Ancient Remedies to Modern Wellness

Introduction:

Essential oils have gained immense popularity in recent years for their aromatic and therapeutic properties. However, the use of essential oils is far from a modern trend. In fact, the history of essential oils dates back thousands of years to ancient civilizations that recognized their remarkable healing potential. In this text, we'll journey through time to explore the rich history of essential oils, from their origins in ancient cultures to their role in modern wellness practices.

Ancient Beginnings:

The use of aromatic plants and their extracts can be traced back to ancient civilizations, including the Egyptians, Greeks, Romans, and Chinese. These early cultures discovered the potent properties of essential oils through trial and error. Here's a glimpse into their ancient practices:

1. Egypt: The Pioneers of Aromatic Oils

Egyptians are often credited as the pioneers of essential oil extraction. They used aromatic oils in religious rituals, cosmetics, and medicine. The famous Ebers Papyrus, dating back to 1550 BCE, contains recipes for various essential oil blends.

2. Greece and Rome: Aromatic Elixirs and Perfumes

Both ancient Greeks and Romans valued the use of aromatic oils. They used essential oils in perfumes, cosmetics, and even as flavorings in food and wine. Hippocrates, the father of modern medicine, incorporated essential oils into his healing treatments.

3. China: Early Herbal Medicine

In ancient China, essential oils were an integral part of Traditional Chinese Medicine (TCM). Aromatics like camphor and cinnamon were used to address various health concerns and balance the body's energies.

Middle Ages: Essential Oils in Europe

During the Middle Ages, the knowledge of essential oils spread to Europe, largely thanks to trade routes with the East. Essential oils were used for their medicinal properties, and they played a crucial role in combating the plagues that swept through Europe.

The Renaissance: Rediscovering Aromatics

The Renaissance period witnessed a resurgence of interest in essential oils. Scholars like Paracelsus explored their medicinal uses, and essential oils became important components of herbal remedies.

19th Century: The Birth of Aromatherapy

The term "aromatherapy" was coined by René-Maurice Gattefossé, a French chemist, in the early 20th century. However, the foundations of aromatherapy were laid in the 19th century when scientists began to study the therapeutic properties of essential oils in more depth.

Modern Revival: Essential Oils Today

In the 21st century, essential oils have experienced a remarkable resurgence in popularity. Their use has expanded beyond traditional medicine to include holistic wellness practices, beauty products, and even household cleaning solutions. With the advent of scientific research, we now have a deeper understanding of the benefits and safety measures associated with essential oils.

Conclusion: Ancient Wisdom for Modern Wellness

The history of essential oils is a testament to the enduring wisdom of ancient cultures. What they discovered through centuries of use, we continue to benefit from today. Whether you're using essential oils for relaxation, skincare, or holistic healing, you're tapping into a tradition that spans millennia. As we blend ancient remedies with modern wellness practices, essential oils remain a fragrant and powerful bridge between our past and our well-being today.

Essential Oils vs. Fragrance Oils: What's the Difference?

Introduction:

When it comes to aromas and scents, many people turn to essential oils and fragrance oils to enhance their surroundings, create personal care products, or simply enjoy pleasant fragrances. While these two types of oils might seem similar, they have distinct differences that affect their origin, composition and uses. In this text, we'll delve into the world of essential and fragrance oils to help you understand the key disparities and make informed choices.

Essential Oils: Nature's Aromatic Essence

1. Sourced from Nature:

Essential oils are natural, aromatic compounds extracted from various parts of plants, such as leaves, flowers, stems, bark, and roots. The extraction methods commonly used include steam distillation, cold pressing, and solvent extraction. These oils capture the essence and fragrance of the plant they are derived from.

2. Complexity of Composition:

Essential oils are composed of numerous chemical compounds, including terpenes, alcohols, esters, and more. These compounds contribute to the unique aroma and therapeutic properties of each oil. Essential oils are known for their complexity and the potential health benefits they offer when used correctly.

3. Therapeutic Properties:

Many essential oils are prized for their therapeutic properties. For example, lavender essential oil is known for its calming effects, while tea tree oil is celebrated for its antibacterial and antifungal properties. These oils can be used in aromatherapy, massage, and as natural remedies for various ailments.

Fragrance Oils: Synthetic Scents for Aesthetics

1. Synthetic Creation:

Fragrance oils, also known as perfume oils or aroma oils, are synthetically created in laboratories. They are designed to mimic the scents of natural substances, such as flowers, fruits, or spices. Fragrance oils are engineered to provide consistent and long-lasting aromas.

2. Simplified Composition:

Compared to essential oils, fragrance oils have a simpler chemical composition. They are typically composed of synthetic aroma chemicals, solvents, and carrier oils. These oils are created to capture a specific scent profile and are often used in perfumes, candles, soaps, and cosmetics.

3. Limited Therapeutic Value:

Fragrance oils are primarily used for their pleasant aroma and are less likely to offer the therapeutic benefits associated with essential oils. While they can enhance the ambiance of a space, they are not typically chosen for their potential health advantages.

Choosing Between Essential Oils and Fragrance Oils:

When deciding between essential and fragrance oils, consider your intended use and goals:

- Aromatherapy and Health Benefits: If you seek therapeutic benefits or intend to use the oils for health-related purposes, essential oils are the better choice.

- Aesthetic and Scent Consistency: If you want a consistent and long-lasting aroma for personal care or home products, fragrance oils may be more suitable.

- Natural vs. Synthetic: Essential oils are natural and plant-based, making them appealing to those who prefer natural products. Fragrance oils are synthetic and offer a wider range of scents.

Conclusion: The Essence of Choice

The choice between essential and fragrance oils ultimately depends on your preferences and needs. While essential oils offer a natural and therapeutic experience, fragrance oils provide a broader range of scents and consistency. Understanding the differences between these two types of oils empowers you to make informed decisions as you explore the aromatic world of oils for your well-being and enjoyment.

Understanding Aromatherapy: How Scents Affect Mood and Health

Introduction:

Aromatherapy, the use of aromatic compounds to enhance well-being, has been practiced for centuries across various cultures. Today, it has gained widespread popularity as a holistic approach to improving mood, reducing stress, and supporting overall health. In this text, we'll delve into the fascinating world of aromatherapy, exploring how scents can have a profound impact on both our mood and physical health.

What Is Aromatherapy?

Aromatherapy is a therapeutic practice that harnesses the power of natural aromatic compounds, primarily essential oils, to promote physical, emotional, and psychological well-being. These aromatic compounds are extracted from plants and have been used for their healing properties for thousands of years.

How Aromatherapy Works: The Sense of Smell

Aromatherapy operates through the olfactory system, which involves our sense of smell. When we inhale the aroma of essential oils, it triggers a complex chain of reactions in our brains.

Here's how it works:

1. Inhalation: When we inhale the scent of essential oils, odor molecules travel through the nasal passages and reach the olfactory bulbs in the brain.

2. Olfactory Bulbs: The olfactory bulbs are responsible for processing scent information. They have direct connections to areas of the brain responsible for emotions and memory, such as the amygdala and the limbic system.

3. Emotional and Physiological Responses: The information processed by the olfactory bulbs can trigger various emotional and physiological responses. This is why certain scents can evoke strong memories or emotions.

Scents and Their Effects on Mood:

Different essential oils are associated with various mood-enhancing properties. Here are a few examples:

1. Lavender: Lavender essential oil is renowned for its calming and relaxing properties. It can reduce stress, anxiety, and improve sleep quality.

2. Citrus Scents: Citrus essential oils like lemon, orange, and grapefruit are invigorating and mood-lifting. They can boost energy and promote a positive outlook.

3. Peppermint: Peppermint essential oil is known for its ability to enhance focus and alertness. It can also relieve headaches and soothe nausea.

4. Eucalyptus: Eucalyptus essential oil has a refreshing and invigorating effect. It can clear the mind and improve respiratory function.

Physical Benefits of Aromatherapy:

In addition to affecting mood, aromatherapy can have tangible physical benefits:

1. Pain Relief: Some essential oils, such as lavender and chamomile, have analgesic properties and can help alleviate pain and muscle tension.

2. Immune Support: Essential oils like tea tree and eucalyptus have antimicrobial properties that can support the immune system.

3. Skin Health: Many essential oils, when diluted properly, can improve skin health by reducing inflammation, acne, and signs of aging.

Aromatherapy Applications:

Aromatherapy can be experienced in various ways:

- Diffusion: Using an essential oil diffuser to disperse scents throughout a room.
- Inhalation: Inhaling essential oil vapors directly or by adding them to hot water.
- Topical Application: Diluting essential oils with carrier oils and applying them to the skin.
- Bath: Adding a few drops of essential oil to a warm bath for relaxation.

Safety Considerations:

While aromatherapy can offer numerous benefits, it's essential to use essential oils safely. Always dilute essential oils before applying them to the skin and be mindful of any allergies or sensitivities.

Conclusion: The Power of Aromatherapy

Aromatherapy is a holistic and natural approach to enhancing mood and promoting well-being. By understanding how scents affect our mood and health, we can harness the power of essential oils to create a more balanced and harmonious life. Whether you're seeking relaxation, increased focus, or relief from physical discomfort, aromatherapy has a scent for you.

Top 10 Must-Have Essential Oils for Beginners

Introduction:

If you're new to the world of essential oils, it can be both exciting and a bit overwhelming to explore the vast array of options available. Essential oils offer a natural and aromatic approach to well-being, and they have a wide range of applications, from relaxation to skincare. To help you start your journey, we've compiled a list of the top 10 must-have essential oils for beginners. These versatile oils are not only easy to use but also offer a variety of benefits that make them essential additions to your collection.

1. Lavender (Lavandula angustifolia): The Universal Oil

Lavender essential oil is often considered the "gateway" oil for beginners. Its soothing aroma promotes relaxation and sleep, making it perfect for stress relief. It also has skin-healing properties and can be used to soothe minor cuts and burns.

2. Peppermint (Mentha × piperita): The Energizer

Peppermint essential oil is invigorating and refreshing. It can help boost energy, improve focus, and relieve headaches. It's also excellent for easing digestive discomfort when diluted and applied topically.

3. Lemon (Citrus limon): The Uplifting Citrus

Lemon essential oil has a bright and cheerful scent that can uplift your mood and improve concentration. It's a natural disinfectant, making it ideal for cleaning and purifying the air.

4. Tea Tree (Melaleuca alternifolia): The Skin Saver

Tea Tree essential oil is well-known for its antiseptic and antibacterial properties. It's an essential addition to your skincare routine, helping with acne, blemishes, and various skin irritations.

5. Eucalyptus (Eucalyptus globulus): The Respiratory Hero

Eucalyptus essential oil is a go-to choice for respiratory support. It can help clear congestion and ease breathing. It's a staple during cold and flu season.

6. Frankincense (Boswellia serrata): The Meditative Oil

Frankincense essential oil has a deep, woody scent that's perfect for meditation and relaxation. It's also known for its skin-rejuvenating properties and is often used in skincare routines.

7. Chamomile (Chamaemelum nobile): The Calming Oil

Chamomile essential oil, particularly Roman chamomile, is soothing and calming. It's great for promoting relaxation, reducing anxiety, and supporting sleep.

8. Rosemary (Rosmarinus officinalis): The Memory Booster

Rosemary essential oil is invigorating and can help improve memory and mental clarity. It's also useful for stimulating hair growth and promoting scalp health.

9. Geranium (Pelargonium graveolens): The Balancer

Geranium essential oil has a balancing effect on emotions and hormones. It's often used to relieve stress, balance the skin's oil production, and reduce inflammation.

10. Cedarwood (Cedrus atlantica): The Grounding Scent

Cedarwood essential oil has a warm and grounding aroma. It's excellent for promoting relaxation, supporting sleep, and soothing skin irritations.

Tips for Beginners:

- Start with a few oils that address your specific needs and interests.

- Always dilute essential oils with a carrier oil when applying to the skin.

- Invest in a quality diffuser to enjoy the aromatic benefits of essential oils.

- Research and learn about each oil's properties and potential uses.

- Experiment with blending oils to create personalized scents and remedies.

Conclusion: Your Essential Journey Begins

These ten essential oils are an excellent starting point for beginners. They offer a broad range of benefits and can be used individually or blended to create custom aromas and remedies. As you explore the world of essential oils, remember to enjoy the journey and discover how these natural wonders can enhance your well-being and daily life.

The Science Behind Essential Oil Extraction Methods

Introduction:

Essential oils are cherished for their aromatic and therapeutic properties, but have you ever wondered how these precious oils are extracted from plants? The science behind essential oil extraction methods is a fascinating journey that involves art, chemistry, and nature. In this text, we'll dive deep into the science behind the extraction of essential oils, exploring various methods used to capture the essence of plants in a bottle.

The Chemistry of Essential Oils: A Complex Symphony

Before delving into extraction methods, it's crucial to understand the chemistry of essential oils. These oils are composed of a wide range of volatile organic compounds, including terpenes, alcohols, esters, and more. It's the unique combination of these compounds that gives each essential oil its distinct aroma and therapeutic properties.

Common Essential Oil Extraction Methods:

1. Steam Distillation:

- Process: In steam distillation, steam is passed through plant material to release the essential oil. The steam and essential oil vapor are then condensed into a liquid.

- Science: Steam carries the volatile compounds from the plant material into the vapor phase. The cooling process condenses the vapor back into liquid, separating the essential oil from the water.

2. Cold Pressing (Expression):

- Process: Cold pressing is primarily used for citrus oils. It involves mechanically pressing the oil from the peel or rind of the fruit.

- Science: The pressure applied ruptures the oil-containing glands in the peel, allowing the essential oil to be released.

3. Solvent Extraction:

- Process: Solvent extraction involves using a solvent (usually hexane) to dissolve the essential oil from the plant material.

- Science: The solvent dissolves the oil, separating it from the plant material. The resulting mixture is then distilled to remove the solvent, leaving behind the essential oil.

4. CO2 Extraction (Supercritical Fluid Extraction):

- Process: CO2 extraction uses carbon dioxide in a supercritical state (neither liquid nor gas) to extract essential oils.

- Science: In its supercritical state, CO_2 acts as a solvent, selectively dissolving the essential oil components. When pressure is reduced, the CO_2 reverts to a gas, leaving behind the extracted essential oil.

5. Hydro-distillation:

- Process: Hydro-distillation is similar to steam distillation but uses water as the solvent instead of steam.

- Science: Water carries essential oil components away from the plant material. The mixture is then separated through the distillation process.

Choosing the Right Method:

The choice of extraction method depends on the plant material, the desired essential oil, and the desired quality. Some methods are more suitable for specific plants, while others preserve the integrity of the oil's chemical composition better.

Quality Matters:

The science of essential oil extraction also emphasizes the importance of quality. Factors like plant source, harvesting techniques, and distillation conditions can all influence the quality of the final product. High-quality oils are typically free from contaminants and possess a well-balanced chemical profile.

Conclusion: Art, Science, and Nature in a Bottle

Essential oil extraction is a harmonious blend of art, science, and nature. The methods employed to capture these aromatic treasures involve a deep understanding of chemistry and a respect for the plant kingdom. Whether it's the steam that carries lavender's soothing essence or the pressure that releases the vibrant scent of citrus, essential oil extraction is a captivating journey into the heart of botanical wonders, all captured in a single drop.

The Power of Inhalation: Using Essential Oils in Diffusers

Introduction:

In the world of aromatherapy, inhalation is a powerful and versatile method for experiencing the benefits of essential oils. Among the various ways to enjoy these natural wonders, using essential oil diffusers is one of the most popular and effective. In this text, we'll explore the fascinating world of diffusing essential oils, highlighting the benefits, types of diffusers, and tips for creating your aromatic oasis at home.

The Science of Inhalation: How It Works

Inhalation is a direct and efficient way to introduce essential oil molecules into your body. When you inhale the aroma of essential oils, the scent molecules travel through the nasal passages and interact with the olfactory receptors. This triggers a cascade of responses in your brain, including the limbic system, which is responsible for emotions and memory. The result? Immediate and profound effects on your mood, emotions, and overall well-being.

Benefits of Diffusing Essential Oils:

1. Stress Reduction: Certain essential oils, like lavender and chamomile, have calming properties that can reduce stress and anxiety.

2. Improved Sleep: Oils like lavender, cedarwood, and bergamot can promote relaxation and improve sleep quality when diffused in the bedroom.

3. Enhanced Focus: Peppermint and rosemary are known to boost concentration and mental clarity, making them great choices for workspaces.

4. Respiratory Support: Eucalyptus, tea tree, and peppermint essential oils can help clear congestion and support respiratory health.

5. Mood Elevation: Citrus oils such as lemon, orange, and grapefruit have uplifting properties that can improve mood and energy levels.

Types of Essential Oil Diffusers:

1. Ultrasonic Diffusers: These diffusers use ultrasonic vibrations to break down essential oils and water into a fine mist. They are gentle on oils and maintain their therapeutic properties. Ultrasonic diffusers also act as humidifiers, adding moisture to the air.

2. Nebulizing Diffusers: Nebulizers disperse essential oils without the use of water, making them potent and highly concentrated. They are ideal for therapeutic purposes but can be intense in smaller spaces.

3. Heat Diffusers: Heat diffusers use heat to evaporate essential oils into the air. While they are simple and affordable, they may alter the chemical composition of the oils and reduce their therapeutic benefits.

4. Evaporative Diffusers: These diffusers use a fan or airflow to evaporate essential oils from a pad or surface. They are cost-effective but may not disperse oils as evenly as other methods.

Tips for Effective Diffusing:

- Use high-quality, pure essential oils for the best results.
- Follow the manufacturer's instructions for your specific diffuser.
- Experiment with oil blends to create personalized aromas.
- Start with a few drops of oil and adjust to your preference.
- Clean your diffuser regularly to prevent oil buildup.

Conclusion: Transform Your Space with Aromatherapy

Using essential oil diffusers is a simple yet powerful way to harness the benefits of aromatherapy in your daily life. Whether you seek relaxation, focus, better sleep, or an uplifting atmosphere, diffusing essential oils can help create the perfect ambiance in your home or workspace. Embrace the world of aromatic possibilities and let the power of inhalation elevate your well-being.

Carrier Oils: The Unsung Heroes of Aromatherapy

Introduction:

When it comes to aromatherapy and essential oil applications, we often hear about the amazing benefits of essential oils themselves. However, there's another essential component in the world of aromatherapy that plays a crucial role in diluting, delivering, and enhancing the effects of essential oils: carrier oils. In this text, we'll shine a light on carrier oils, exploring their significance, types, and how they contribute to the safe and effective use of essential oils.

What Are Carrier Oils?

Carrier oils, also known as base oils or vegetable oils, are neutral, non-volatile oils extracted from various plant sources, such as seeds, nuts, and fruits. Unlike essential oils, which are highly concentrated and aromatic, carrier oils have a mild aroma and serve as a vehicle for diluting and dispersing essential oils for topical use.

The Significance of Carrier Oils:

1. Dilution: Essential oils are potent and can cause skin irritation when applied undiluted. Carrier oils are used to dilute essential oils, making them safer for topical application.

2. Aromatic Enhancement: Carrier oils help slow down the evaporation of essential oils, allowing their aromas to be released more gradually and last longer when applied to the skin.

3. Skin Nourishment: Carrier oils are rich in fatty acids, vitamins, and minerals that provide nourishment and hydration to the skin. They can improve skin texture and act as natural moisturizers.

Popular Carrier Oils and Their Benefits:

1. Jojoba Oil: Jojoba oil closely resembles the skin's natural sebum and is easily absorbed. It's excellent for facial care and is suitable for all skin types.

2. Coconut Oil: Coconut oil is hydrating and has antimicrobial properties. It's a popular choice for massage and hair treatments.

3. Sweet Almond Oil: Rich in vitamin E and fatty acids, sweet almond oil is nourishing and soothing to the skin. It's suitable for sensitive skin.

4. Grapeseed Oil: Grapeseed oil is lightweight and absorbs quickly. It's known for its astringent properties and is often used in skincare products.

5. Olive Oil: Olive oil is a versatile carrier oil with antioxidant properties. It's great for massage and can be used in hair care.

How to Use Carrier Oils with Essential Oils:

- To create a diluted essential oil blend, mix a few drops of essential oil with a carrier oil. The ratio depends on the oil's purpose and the individual's sensitivity, typically ranging from 1% to 5% essential oil concentration.

- Carrier oils can be used as massage oils, body oils, or as a base for making natural skincare products like creams and lotions.

- They can also be used for oil cleansing, a method to remove makeup and cleanse the skin using natural oils.

Conclusion: Carrier Oils, the Unsung Support

Carrier oils may not steal the spotlight, but they play a vital role in the world of aromatherapy. They provide a safe and nourishing medium for essential oils to work their magic while offering their benefits to the skin. As you embark on your aromatherapy journey, don't underestimate the importance of carrier oils in enhancing your well-being and ensuring a pleasant and effective aromatic experience. These unsung heroes are essential companions on the path to holistic health and natural beauty.

DIY Essential Oil Blending: Creating Your Signature Scent

Introduction:

There's something truly magical about crafting your own signature scent using essential oils. DIY essential oil blending allows you to combine your favorite aromatic notes to create a unique fragrance that resonates with your personality and preferences. In this text, we'll guide you through the art of essential oil blending, providing tips, recipes, and inspiration to help you craft your very own bespoke fragrance.

The Art of Essential Oil Blending:

Blending essential oils is both an art and a science. It involves combining different essential oils in precise ratios to achieve a balanced aroma that suits your taste. Here's how to get started:

1. Gather Your Essential Oils:

Begin by selecting a variety of essential oils with scents that resonate with you. Consider top, middle, and base notes:

- Top Notes: These are the first scents you'll notice and typically include citrus and herbal oils like lemon, lavender, and peppermint.

- Middle Notes: These provide depth and balance to the fragrance and include floral and spicy oils like rose, chamomile, and geranium.

- Base Notes: These are the foundation of the scent and include woody, earthy, and resinous oils like cedarwood, patchouli, and frankincense.

2. Understand Scent Profiles:

To create a harmonious blend, it's essential to understand scent profiles. Blends often consist of a combination of top, middle, and base notes to create a balanced and long-lasting fragrance.

3. Experiment with Ratios:

Start with small quantities and experiment with different ratios of essential oils. A common ratio for a balanced blend is 30% top notes, 50% middle notes, and 20% base notes. Adjust these ratios based on your preference.

4. Keep Notes:

As you blend, keep a journal of your recipes and the ratios used. This will help you recreate your favorite blends in the future.

DIY Essential Oil Blending Recipes:

Here are a few simple essential oil blend recipes to get you started:

1. Citrus Splash:

- 3 drops of lemon (top note)
- 3 drops of sweet orange (top note)
- 2 drops of lavender (middle note)

2. Floral Breeze:

- 4 drops of lavender (middle note)
- 3 drops of rose (middle note)
- 2 drops of ylang-ylang (middle note)

3. Woodsy Serenity:

- 3 drops of cedarwood (base note)
- 2 drops of frankincense (base note)
- 2 drops of lavender (middle note)

Tips for Blending Success:

- Start with a small batch to avoid wasting essential oils.

- Use a glass bottle to store your blend, as plastic can interact with the oils.

- Allow your blend to mature for a few days to a week, as the scent may change and evolve over time.

Conclusion: A Fragrant Journey of Self-Expression

Creating your own signature scent through DIY essential oil blending is a delightful journey of self-expression. With patience and creativity, you can craft fragrances that resonate with your unique personality and bring joy to your daily life. So, gather your essential oils, experiment with different combinations, and let your creativity flow as you embark on this aromatic adventure. Your signature scent awaits, ready to captivate your senses and those around you.

Essential Oils for Skin: Tips for Safe and Effective Application

Introduction:

Essential oils have gained immense popularity for their natural and holistic approach to skincare. When used correctly, essential oils can offer a wide range of benefits, from promoting skin health to addressing specific concerns. However, it's crucial to understand how to use them safely and effectively to maximize their potential without causing harm. In this text, we'll explore essential oils for skin, providing tips and guidelines for safe and effective application.

1. Choose High-Quality Essential Oils:

The quality of essential oils matters. Look for oils that are 100% pure and free from synthetic additives or contaminants. Reputable brands often provide information about their sourcing, extraction methods, and testing processes.

2. Dilute Essential Oils:

Essential oils are highly concentrated and can be potent, which is why they should be diluted before applying them to the skin. Always use carrier oil, such as jojoba, sweet almond, or coconut oil, to dilute essential oils. A common dilution ratio is 2-3 drops of essential oil per teaspoon of carrier oil.

3. Patch Test:

Before applying an essential oil blend to a larger area of your skin, perform a patch test. Apply a small amount of the diluted blend to the inside of your wrist or forearm. Wait 24 hours to check for any adverse reactions like redness, itching, or irritation.

4. Be Cautious with Sensitizing Oils:

Some essential oils, like cinnamon, clove, and oregano, are known as sensitizing oils and can cause skin irritation even when diluted. Use them sparingly and with caution.

5. Sun Sensitivity:

Certain citrus essential oils, such as bergamot and lime, can make your skin more sensitive to UV rays. Avoid direct sun exposure after applying these oils to your skin, or use them in the evening.

6. Targeted Applications:

Essential oils can be used for targeted applications, such as spot treatments for acne or scars. Apply a small amount directly to the affected area using a clean fingertip or a cotton swab.

7. Facial Steam:

For a spa-like experience, add a few drops of essential oil to a bowl of hot water, cover your head with a towel, and inhale the steam. This can help cleanse and rejuvenate your skin.

8. Customize Your Skincare:

Consider incorporating essential oils into your existing skincare routine. You can add a few drops to your facial cleanser, moisturizer, or even your bath for an aromatic experience.

9. Store Essential Oils Properly:

Keep your essential oils in dark glass bottles, away from direct sunlight and heat. Store them in a cool, dry place to preserve their potency.

10. Listen to Your Skin:

Pay attention to how your skin responds to essential oils. If you experience any discomfort or adverse reactions, discontinue use immediately. Not all essential oils are suitable for all skin types, so it's important to find what works best for you.

Conclusion: The Art of Nurturing Your Skin Naturally

Essential oils can be excellent allies in your skincare journey when used mindfully and responsibly. By following these tips and guidelines for safe and practical application, you can harness the power of essential oils to support your skin's health and well-being. Embrace the art of nurturing your skin naturally and enjoy the benefits of radiant, refreshed, and rejuvenated skin.

The Role of Essential Oils in Traditional Chinese Medicine

Introduction:

Traditional Chinese Medicine (TCM) is a holistic system of healing that has been practiced for thousands of years. It encompasses various modalities, including acupuncture, herbal medicine, cupping therapy, and qigong. While not as well-known as other aspects of TCM, essential oils have also played a significant role in this ancient healing tradition. In this text, we'll explore the fascinating connection between essential oils and Traditional Chinese Medicine, shedding light on their history, applications, and therapeutic benefits.

Essential Oils in Traditional Chinese Medicine: A Historical Perspective

The use of essential oils in TCM can be traced back over 2,000 years. Ancient texts like the Huangdi Neijing (Yellow Emperor's Inner Canon) mention the use of aromatic substances for healing and balancing the body's energy. Essential oils, derived from plants and their aromatic parts, were considered powerful tools for influencing the flow of qi (energy) and promoting harmony within the body.

Key Concepts in TCM and Essential Oils:

1. Five Elements Theory: TCM is based on the concept of five elements (Wood, Fire, Earth, Metal, Water) and their correspondences with various aspects of the body and emotions. Certain essential oils are associated with these elements and can be used to balance them. For example, wood element oils like cedarwood and tea tree can support the liver and gallbladder meridians.

2. Meridian System: TCM identifies a network of meridians through which qi flows. Each meridian is associated with specific organs and functions. Essential oils can be applied to acupoints along these meridians to influence the flow of qi and promote balance.

3. Yin and Yang: TCM emphasizes the balance between yin (cooling, passive) and yang (warming, active) energies in the body. Essential oils are categorized as yin or yang based on their properties and can be used to harmonize these opposing forces.

Applications of Essential Oils in TCM:

1. Aromatherapy: Essential oils are used in TCM aromatherapy to influence the mind and emotions. Oils like lavender, rose, and frankincense are often employed to calm the spirit and ease emotional imbalances.

2. Topical Applications: Essential oils are diluted with carrier oils and applied to specific acupoints or meridians to address physical and emotional issues. For example, peppermint oil can be applied to acupoints on the head to relieve headaches.

3. Moxibustion: Moxibustion is a TCM therapy involving the burning of dried mugwort (moxa) near acupoints to stimulate qi flow. Essential oils can enhance the therapeutic effects of moxibustion by adding their aromatic properties to the treatment.

Safety and Precautions:

- Always dilute essential oils before applying them to the skin.
- Consult with a qualified TCM practitioner or aromatherapist who is knowledgeable about TCM before using essential oils for specific health concerns.
- Be mindful of individual sensitivities and allergies when using essential oils.

Conclusion: Bridging Ancient Wisdom with Modern Wellness

The integration of essential oils into Traditional Chinese Medicine represents a harmonious blend of ancient wisdom and modern wellness practices. These aromatic treasures offer a holistic approach to healing and balance by influencing the body's energy flow, emotions, and overall well-being. By understanding the principles of TCM and essential oils, individuals can explore the therapeutic benefits of this ancient tradition and enhance their journey toward health and harmony.

Aromatherapy for Stress Relief: Managing Everyday Tensions

Introduction:

In today's fast-paced world, stress has become a common companion in our daily lives. Whether it's work-related pressure, personal challenges, or the demands of modern living, stress can take a toll on our well-being. Aromatherapy, the use of essential oils for therapeutic purposes, offers a natural and effective way to manage everyday tensions and promote relaxation. In this text, we'll explore how aromatherapy can be a powerful tool for stress relief and share tips for incorporating it into your self-care routine.

Understanding Stress and Its Impact:

Stress is a natural response to challenging situations, but chronic stress can have adverse effects on our physical and mental health. It can lead to symptoms like anxiety, tension, headaches, and sleep disturbances. Finding healthy ways to manage stress is essential for overall well-being.

Aromatherapy as a Stress Management Tool:

Aromatherapy utilizes the aromatic compounds of essential oils to promote relaxation, reduce anxiety, and alleviate stress-related symptoms. Here's how it works:

1. Affects the Limbic System: When we inhale the aroma of essential oils, the scent molecules stimulate the olfactory receptors in our nose. These receptors send signals to the limbic system, the part of the brain responsible for emotions and memory. This connection allows essential oils to influence our mood and emotional well-being.

2. Balances the Autonomic Nervous System: Aromatherapy can help regulate the autonomic nervous system, which controls our body's stress response. Certain essential oils have a calming effect, promoting the parasympathetic (relaxation) response and reducing the sympathetic (fight-or-flight) response.

Essential Oils for Stress Relief:

1. Lavender (Lavandula angustifolia): Lavender is renowned for its calming properties. Its gentle and soothing aroma helps reduce anxiety and promote relaxation. It's excellent for bedtime or when you need to unwind.

2. Chamomile (Chamaemelum nobile): Chamomile essential oil has a calming and comforting scent. It's particularly beneficial for easing tension and promoting relaxation.

3. Bergamot (Citrus bergamia): Bergamot oil has a delightful citrus aroma that can uplift the mood and reduce stress and anxiety. It's a great choice for daytime use.

4. Frankincense (Boswellia serrata): Frankincense essential oil is grounding and meditative. It can help alleviate stress and promote a sense of inner peace and tranquility.

5. Ylang-Ylang (Cananga odorata): Ylang-ylang has a sweet, exotic fragrance that is known for its ability to reduce stress and promote a sense of well-being.

Incorporating Aromatherapy into Your Routine:

- Diffusers: Use an essential oil diffuser to disperse the aroma of your chosen oil throughout your home or workspace.

- Inhalation: Inhale the scent directly from the bottle or apply a drop to a tissue or cotton ball for on-the-go stress relief.

- Baths: Add a few drops of essential oil to your bathwater for a relaxing soak.

- Massage: Dilute the essential oil in a carrier oil and use it for a stress-relieving massage.

- DIY Blends: Experiment with creating your own blends of essential oils to find the combination that works best for you.

Conclusion: A Calming Refuge in Aromatherapy

Aromatherapy offers a gentle and natural approach to managing everyday stress. By harnessing the power of essential oils, you can create a calming refuge in your daily life, promoting relaxation, emotional balance, and overall well-being. Whether you prefer the soothing scent of lavender or the uplifting aroma of bergamot, there's an essential oil waiting to help you manage life's tensions and find your inner calm.

The Antimicrobial Properties of Essential Oils

Introduction:

In an era where antimicrobial resistance is a growing concern, nature has provided us with a powerful ally: essential oils. These aromatic extracts, derived from plants, have been used for centuries not only for their captivating scents but also for their remarkable antimicrobial properties. In this text, we'll delve into the world of essential oils and explore how they can serve as effective natural alternatives to conventional antimicrobial agents.

The Power of Essential Oils:

Essential oils are concentrated liquids extracted from various parts of plants, including leaves, flowers, bark, and roots. They contain a complex mixture of volatile compounds, each with its own unique therapeutic properties. Among these properties, their ability to combat microbes has gained increasing attention from researchers and health enthusiasts alike.

Antimicrobial Agents in Essential Oils:

1. Terpenes: Terpenes are a class of compounds commonly found in essential oils. Many terpenes exhibit antimicrobial activity. For

example, limonene, found in citrus oils like lemon and orange, has been shown to have antibacterial properties.

2. Phenols: Phenolic compounds, such as thymol and carvacrol found in oregano and thyme oils, possess potent antimicrobial properties. They can disrupt the cell membranes of bacteria, rendering them inactive.

3. Aldehydes: Essential oils like cinnamon and lemongrass contain aldehydes like cinnamaldehyde and citronellal, which have strong antimicrobial effects.

4. Monoterpenoids: Monoterpenoids found in oils like tea tree and eucalyptus, such as terpinen-4-ol, are known for their antimicrobial and antifungal properties.

Applications of Essential Oils as Antimicrobials:

1. Hand Sanitizers: Many commercial hand sanitizers contain synthetic antimicrobial agents. Essential oils like tea tree, lavender, and thyme can be used to create natural hand sanitizers that are just as effective.

2. Surface Disinfectants: Essential oils can be added to homemade cleaning solutions to create natural disinfectants for countertops, floors, and other surfaces.

3. Oral Health: Some essential oils, such as clove and peppermint, can be used as mouthwashes to combat oral bacteria and promote fresh breath.

4. Skin Infections: Tea tree oil, with its strong antimicrobial properties, is often used topically to treat skin infections, acne, and minor cuts and scrapes.

5. Respiratory Health: Inhalation of essential oils like eucalyptus and thyme can help alleviate respiratory infections and congestion.

Safety and Precautions:

While essential oils can be potent antimicrobial agents, they should be used with care:

- Always dilute essential oils before applying them to the skin or using them in cleaning products.
- Conduct a patch test to check for any skin sensitivities or allergies.
- Some essential oils are not safe for internal use, so consult with a qualified aromatherapist or healthcare practitioner before ingesting them.
- Keep essential oils out of reach of children and pets.

Conclusion: Nature's Gift for a Healthier World

Essential oils offer a natural and effective way to harness the antimicrobial power of plants. Whether you're seeking a natural alternative to commercial sanitizers, a way to freshen your home without harsh chemicals, or a remedy for common skin issues, essential oils can be valuable allies in your journey toward a healthier, more sustainable lifestyle. As we navigate the challenges of antimicrobial resistance, nature's gifts in the form of essential oils remind us of the powerful solutions that lie at our fingertips.

Essential Oils and Chakras: Balancing Energy Centers

Introduction:

The concept of chakras, originating from ancient Indian traditions, has gained popularity in holistic wellness practices worldwide. Chakras are believed to be spinning energy centers within the body, each associated with specific physical, emotional, and spiritual attributes. Essential oils, with their unique aromatic and therapeutic properties, can play a significant role in balancing and harmonizing these chakras. We'll explore the connection between essential oils and chakras, delving into each energy center and the oils that can help balance them.

Understanding Chakras:

Chakras are often depicted as spinning wheels or vortexes of energy located along the central axis of the body. There are seven primary chakras, each associated with a specific color, element, sound, and aspect of our being:

1. Root Chakra (Muladhara): Located at the base of the spine, the root chakra is associated with stability, grounding, and the element of Earth.

2. Sacral Chakra (Svadhisthana): Positioned in the lower abdomen, the sacral chakra relates to creativity, sexuality, and the element of Water.

3. Solar Plexus Chakra (Manipura): Found in the upper abdomen, the solar plexus chakra governs personal power, confidence, and the element of Fire.

4. Heart Chakra (Anahata): Centered in the chest, the heart chakra is associated with love, compassion, and the element of Air.

5. Throat Chakra (Vishuddha): Located at the throat, the throat chakra is linked to communication, self-expression, and the element of Sound.

6. Third Eye Chakra (Ajna): Positioned in the forehead between the eyebrows, the third eye chakra is associated with intuition, insight, and the element of Light.

7. Crown Chakra (Sahasrara): Located at the crown of the head, the crown chakra represents spiritual connection, enlightenment, and the element of Thought.

Using Essential Oils for Chakra Balancing:

Essential oils, with their diverse aromatic profiles and healing properties, can be used to balance and activate the chakras. Here's a breakdown of each chakra and the corresponding essential oils:

1. Root Chakra (Muladhara):
   - Essential Oils: Cedarwood, Patchouli, Vetiver
   - Benefits: Grounding, stability, security

2. Sacral Chakra (Svadhisthana):
   - Essential Oils: Sweet Orange, Ylang-Ylang, Sandalwood
   - Benefits: Creativity, emotional balance, sensuality

3. Solar Plexus Chakra (Manipura):
   - Essential Oils: Lemon, Peppermint, Ginger
   - Benefits: Confidence, self-esteem, empowerment

4. Heart Chakra (Anahata):
   - Essential Oils: Rose, Lavender, Bergamot
   - Benefits: Love, compassion, healing

5. Throat Chakra (Vishuddha):
   - Essential Oils: Eucalyptus, Spearmint, Chamomile
   - Benefits: Communication, self-expression, truth

6. Third Eye Chakra (Ajna):
   - Essential Oils: Frankincense, Lavender, Clary Sage

- Benefits: Intuition, insight, clarity

7. Crown Chakra (Sahasrara):

  - Essential Oils: Lavender, Frankincense, Myrrh

  - Benefits: Spiritual connection, enlightenment, higher consciousness

How to Use Essential Oils for Chakra Balancing:

- Diffusion: Add a few drops of the appropriate essential oil to a diffuser during meditation or relaxation practices.

- Topical Application: Dilute essential oils with a carrier oil and apply them to the chakra area during chakra-balancing rituals or massage.

- Aromatherapy Jewelry: Wear diffuser jewelry to carry the aroma of specific essential oils with you throughout the day.

- Chakra Roll-Ons: Create or purchase pre-diluted chakra roll-on blends for convenient and targeted applications.

Conclusion: Aligning Body, Mind, and Spirit

Balancing your chakras with essential oils can be a transformative journey toward greater well-being and self-awareness. By incorporating the aromatic and therapeutic qualities of essential oils into your chakra-balancing practices, you can align your energy centers, promote emotional harmony, and enhance your spiritual connection. Whether you're a seasoned practitioner or new to chakra work, the world of essential oils offers a delightful and effective way to nurture your body, mind, and spirit, bringing you closer to holistic balance and well-being.

Aromatherapy for Pets: Enhancing Your Pet's Well-Being

Introduction:

Aromatherapy, long appreciated for its therapeutic benefits in humans, is gaining recognition as a valuable tool for enhancing the well-being of our beloved pets. Just as essential oils can promote relaxation, alleviate stress, and address various physical and emotional issues in humans, they can offer similar benefits to our furry companions. In this comprehensive text, we'll explore the world of aromatherapy for pets, covering its safety, potential benefits, and practical applications to help you support your pet's health and happiness.

Understanding Aromatherapy for Pets:

Aromatherapy for pets involves the use of essential oils, which are concentrated extracts from aromatic plants, to promote physical and emotional balance in animals. These essential oils can be diffused, applied topically, or incorporated into various pet care routines to address specific concerns or enhance overall well-being.

Safety Considerations:

Before we delve into the potential benefits of aromatherapy for pets, it's essential to emphasize safety:

1. Dilution: Essential oils must always be diluted before use on pets. Dilute them with a carrier oil to avoid skin irritation.

2. Selection: Not all essential oils are safe for pets. Some oils can be toxic to dogs, cats, or other animals. Consult with a veterinarian or experienced aromatherapist to ensure you choose pet-safe oils.

3. Dosage: Use essential oils sparingly and in appropriate quantities for your pet's size and species. Less is often more when it comes to aromatherapy for pets.

4. Observation: Pay close attention to your pet's reaction when introducing aromatherapy. If you notice any adverse effects, discontinue use immediately.

Potential Benefits of Aromatherapy for Pets:

1. Stress Reduction: Aromatherapy can help alleviate stress and anxiety in pets, particularly during thunderstorms, fireworks, or other stressful situations.

2. Pain Relief: Certain essential oils, when used under professional guidance, can offer pain relief for pets dealing with arthritis or other chronic conditions.

3. Improved Sleep: Aromatic blends can create a calming atmosphere that promotes restful sleep for pets.

4. Enhanced Focus: Aromatherapy can aid in training and behavior modification by helping pets stay focused and relaxed.

5. Skin and Coat Health: Some oils, when diluted correctly, can promote skin and coat health and address common issues like itching and inflammation.

Practical Applications:

1. Diffusion: Use a pet-safe essential oil diffuser to create a calming atmosphere in your home. Oils like lavender and chamomile can be particularly soothing.

2. Topical Application: Dilute essential oils in a carrier oil and apply them to your pet's collar, bedding, or a bandana for lasting aromatherapy benefits.

3. Massage: Gentle massages using diluted essential oils can promote relaxation and alleviate muscle tension.

4. Bath Time: Incorporate pet-safe essential oils into your pet's bath routine to address skin issues or simply make bath time a more pleasant experience.

Pet-Safe Essential Oils:

- For dogs: Lavender, chamomile, cedarwood, and frankincense are generally safe when diluted properly.

- For cats: Be cautious with essential oils around cats, as their liver metabolizes compounds differently. Consult a veterinarian for safe options.

- For other animals: Always consult with a veterinarian or experienced aromatherapist to ensure the safety of essential oil use for pets other than dogs and cats.

Conclusion: Nurturing Your Pet's Wellness Naturally

Aromatherapy for pets offers a natural and gentle way to enhance the well-being of your furry friends. When used thoughtfully and safely, essential oils can be a valuable addition to your pet care routine. By understanding the principles of aromatherapy and seeking guidance when needed, you can nurture your pet's wellness naturally, creating a harmonious and happy environment that supports their physical and emotional health. Remember that the well-being of your pet should always be the top priority, and consulting with a veterinarian or professional aromatherapist is essential for the safe and effective use of aromatherapy.

Essential Oils for Men's Health: From Beard Care to Libido Boosting

Introduction:

Essential oils, long celebrated for their therapeutic properties, are increasingly gaining recognition as versatile tools for men's health and well-being. Whether it's taming a magnificent beard, relieving stress, or enhancing vitality, essential oils offer a wide array of benefits tailored to men's unique needs. In this comprehensive text, we'll explore the world of essential oils for men's health, covering grooming tips, stress relief strategies, and natural approaches to boost vitality.

Essential Oils for Beard Care:

1. Tea Tree (Melaleuca alternifolia): Tea tree oil helps prevent beard dandruff and skin irritation. It has natural antifungal and antibacterial properties that keep the skin beneath the beard healthy.

2. Jojoba (Simmondsia chinensis): Jojoba oil is an excellent carrier oil for beard oils and balms. It closely resembles the skin's natural oils, making it an ideal choice for moisturizing and conditioning the beard.

3. Peppermint (Mentha × piperita): Peppermint oil adds a refreshing scent to beard care products. Its invigorating aroma can also help improve focus and concentration during grooming.

Stress Relief and Relaxation:

1. Lavender (Lavandula angustifolia): Lavender oil is renowned for its calming properties. It can help reduce stress, promote relaxation, and improve sleep quality.

2. Frankincense (Boswellia serrata): Frankincense essential oil has a grounding aroma that can ease anxiety and create a sense of inner peace.

3. Cedarwood (Cedrus atlantica): Cedarwood oil is known for its calming effects. It can help alleviate tension and promote relaxation after a long day.

Energy and Vitality:

1. Black Pepper (Piper nigrum): Black pepper oil has a warming and invigorating scent that can help boost energy levels and enhance mental alertness.

2. Ginger (Zingiber officinale): Ginger oil is energizing and can help improve circulation, making it a valuable addition to massage blends.

3. Rosemary (Rosmarinus officinalis): Rosemary essential oil has a stimulating aroma that can increase focus and mental clarity.

Libido and Vitality:

1. Sandalwood (Santalum album): Sandalwood oil is often used to enhance mood and libido. Its rich, woody scent is both relaxing and arousing.

2. Ylang-Ylang (Cananga odorata): Ylang-ylang oil has a sensual fragrance that can boost confidence and enhance desire.

3. Ginseng (Panax ginseng): Ginseng oil, when used sparingly and under professional guidance, is believed to support vitality and stamina.

Practical Applications:

1. Beard Oils: Create your own beard oil blend by mixing carrier oils like jojoba and argan with a few drops of essential oils for a well-groomed and healthy beard.

2. Diffusion: Use an essential oil diffuser to fill your space with invigorating or relaxing scents, depending on your mood and needs.

3. Massage: Incorporate essential oils into massage oils or lotions for a soothing and revitalizing experience.

4. Aromatherapy Inhalers: Create portable inhalers with essential oils to boost focus, relieve stress, or enhance vitality throughout the day.

Safety Considerations:

- Always dilute essential oils before applying them to the skin.
- Conduct a patch test to check for any skin sensitivities or allergies.
- Use essential oils sparingly and in moderation, as some can be quite potent.

Conclusion: Nurturing Men's Health Naturally

Essential oils offer a natural and effective way to support men's health and well-being, from grooming to stress relief and vitality. By incorporating these aromatic treasures into your daily routine, you can harness their therapeutic benefits and enjoy a more balanced and vibrant life. Remember to prioritize safety and consult with a qualified aromatherapist or healthcare professional when needed to make the most of essential oils for your specific health goals.

The Benefits of Steam Inhalation with Essential Oils

Introduction:

Steam inhalation with essential oils is a centuries-old practice that offers a wide range of therapeutic benefits for the respiratory system, skin, and overall well-being. Whether you're seeking relief from congestion, stress reduction, or a natural skincare remedy, steam inhalation can be a simple yet powerful addition to your self-care routine. In this comprehensive text, we'll explore the art of steam inhalation with essential oils, its history, benefits, and practical applications.

The Ancient Practice of Steam Inhalation:

Steam inhalation, also known as steam therapy or aromatherapy steam, has roots in ancient healing traditions. Throughout history, various cultures have used the inhalation of steam infused with herbs and aromatic substances to promote health and alleviate discomfort.

How Steam Inhalation Works:

Steam inhalation involves the use of steam to disperse the volatile compounds of essential oils into the air. When inhaled, these aromatic molecules interact with our olfactory system and respiratory tract, delivering a range of therapeutic effects. Here's how it works:

1. Opening Air Passages: The warm steam helps open nasal passages and airways, making it easier to breathe and relieving congestion.

2. Aromatic Inhalation: As you breathe in the steam, the essential oil molecules are carried deep into the respiratory system, where they can have a direct impact on the body.

Benefits of Steam Inhalation with Essential Oils:

1. Respiratory Relief: Steam inhalation can provide quick relief from nasal congestion, sinusitis, and respiratory discomfort associated with colds and allergies.

2. Stress Reduction: Aromatherapy steam can help calm the mind, reduce stress, and promote relaxation, making it a valuable addition to relaxation practices.

3. Skin Health: Steam opens pores, allowing essential oils to penetrate the skin, making it an effective treatment for acne, dry skin, and overall skin health.

4. Mental Clarity: Certain essential oils used in steam inhalation, such as eucalyptus and rosemary, can enhance mental clarity, focus, and alertness.

Popular Essential Oils for Steam Inhalation:

1. Eucalyptus (Eucalyptus globulus): Eucalyptus oil is excellent for respiratory support and clearing congestion.

2. Lavender (Lavandula angustifolia): Lavender's calming aroma is perfect for relaxation and stress relief.

3. Peppermint (Mentha × piperita): Peppermint oil offers invigorating and cooling properties, ideal for mental alertness.

4. Tea Tree (Melaleuca alternifolia): Tea tree oil has antibacterial properties and is beneficial for skin health.

Practical Applications:

1. Facial Steam: To promote clear and healthy skin, add a few drops of essential oil to a bowl of steaming water. Lean over the bowl with a towel covering your head to trap the steam and inhale deeply.

2. Inhaler Sticks: Portable inhaler sticks can be pre-loaded with essential oils for on-the-go relief.

3. Shower Aromatherapy: Place a few drops of essential oil on a wet washcloth and hang it in the shower for a spa-like experience.

4. Diffuser with Steam Function: Some diffusers have a steam function that combines essential oil diffusion with steam, creating a soothing atmosphere.

Safety Considerations:

- Always dilute essential oils before using them in steam inhalation, as undiluted oils can be too strong and potentially irritate the skin or respiratory tract.
- Be cautious with the temperature of the steam to avoid burns.
- Keep your eyes closed during steam inhalation to prevent irritation.

Conclusion: A Breath of Wellness

Steam inhalation with essential oils offers a breath of wellness for both the body and the mind. Whether you're seeking relief from respiratory discomfort, relaxation, or an effective skincare treatment, this ancient practice can be a valuable addition to your self-care routine. By exploring the aromatic wonders of essential oils through steam inhalation, you can harness the healing power of nature in the comfort of your own home. Remember to prioritize safety and consult a qualified aromatherapist for personalized guidance on essential oil selection and usage.

Aromatherapy Jewelry: Wearable Wellness

Introduction:

Aromatherapy, the practice of using essential oils for therapeutic benefits, has found a fashionable and portable companion in aromatherapy jewelry. These beautifully crafted accessories offer a stylish way to carry the soothing scents of essential oils with you throughout the day, providing both aesthetic appeal and wellness benefits. In this comprehensive text, we'll explore the world of aromatherapy jewelry, its history, types, benefits, and how to use it to enhance your well-being.

The Art and History of Aromatherapy Jewelry:

Aromatherapy jewelry combines the ancient practice of using aromatic substances for healing with contemporary fashion sensibilities. These jewelry pieces are designed to hold essential oils and diffuse their fragrances gradually, allowing you to enjoy the therapeutic effects of aromatherapy wherever you go.

Types of Aromatherapy Jewelry:

1. Aromatherapy Necklaces: These necklaces often feature a pendant that holds a small piece of absorbent material, such as a felt pad or lava stone, where you can apply a few drops of essential oil.

2. Aromatherapy Bracelets: Aromatherapy bracelets typically have porous beads, stones, or wooden elements that can hold and release the aroma of essential oils.

3. Aromatherapy Earrings: Some earrings have tiny diffuser compartments where you can place essential oil-infused materials.

4. Aromatherapy Rings: These rings may contain small chambers for essential oil application, allowing you to enjoy the scents discreetly.

Benefits of Aromatherapy Jewelry:

1. Stress Reduction: Aromatherapy jewelry can provide on-the-go stress relief and relaxation, helping you stay calm and centered throughout the day.

2. Mood Enhancement: Certain essential oils, like citrus oils, can uplift your mood when diffused through aromatherapy jewelry.

3. Focus and Concentration: Aromatherapy can aid in enhancing mental clarity and concentration, making it a valuable tool for work or study.

4. Personalized Aromatherapy: Aromatherapy jewelry allows you to choose the essential oils that suit your needs and preferences, tailoring your wellness experience.

Using Aromatherapy Jewelry:

1. Select Your Essential Oils: Choose essential oils that align with your desired outcome, whether it's relaxation, energy, or stress relief.

2. Apply the Oil: Place a drop or two of your chosen essential oil onto the absorbent material or beads of the jewelry. Allow the oil to be absorbed before wearing it.

3. Enjoy the Aroma: Wear your aromatherapy jewelry throughout the day, and gently inhale the scent whenever you need a wellness boost.

4. Reapply as Needed: Essential oils may evaporate or lose their scent over time. Reapply as needed to maintain the aroma.

Cleaning and Maintenance:

To keep your aromatherapy jewelry in optimal condition:

- Clean the jewelry regularly to prevent oil buildup.
- Use a mild soap and water solution to clean the jewelry, avoiding harsh chemicals gently.
- Allow the jewelry to air dry thoroughly before reapplying essential oils.

Conclusion: Style Meets Wellness

Aromatherapy jewelry seamlessly blends style with wellness, offering a fashionable and convenient way to experience the benefits of essential oils. Whether you're seeking relaxation, stress relief, or a mood boost, these beautifully designed accessories provide a personalized and discreet aromatherapy experience.

By embracing the world of aromatherapy jewelry, you can carry the scents of nature with you, enhancing your well-being and style simultaneously. Enjoy the fusion of fashion and wellness with aromatherapy jewelry, and make it an integral part of your daily self-care routine.

Essential Oils for Seasonal Allergies: Natural Relief

Introduction:

Seasonal allergies, often triggered by pollen, grass, and other environmental factors, can be a source of discomfort for many people. While over-the-counter medications are commonly used to alleviate symptoms, essential oils offer a natural and holistic approach to finding relief from sneezing, congestion, and itchy eyes. In this comprehensive text, we'll explore the world of essential oils for seasonal allergies, including their benefits, application methods, and popular oil choices to help you breathe easier and enjoy the changing seasons.

Understanding Seasonal Allergies:

Seasonal allergies, also known as hay fever or allergic rhinitis, occur when the immune system reacts to allergens in the environment. Common symptoms include sneezing, congestion, runny nose, itchy eyes, and coughing. While allergies can be managed with conventional medication, essential oils offer a natural alternative for relief.

Benefits of Essential Oils for Seasonal Allergies:

1. Anti-Inflammatory: Some essential oils have natural anti-inflammatory properties that can help reduce nasal inflammation and congestion.

2. Antihistamine Effect: Certain oils may have antihistamine-like effects, which can alleviate allergy symptoms triggered by histamine release.

3. Decongestant: Essential oils with decongestant properties can help open airways and improve breathing.

4. Relaxation: Aromatherapy with soothing oils can help reduce stress and promote overall well-being, which may complement allergy relief.

Popular Essential Oils for Seasonal Allergies:

1. Lavender (Lavandula angustifolia): Lavender oil has anti-inflammatory and calming properties, making it a valuable choice for relieving allergy symptoms and promoting relaxation.

2. Peppermint (Mentha × piperita): Peppermint oil acts as a natural decongestant and can help clear nasal passages.

3. Eucalyptus (Eucalyptus globulus): Eucalyptus oil has both anti-inflammatory and decongestant properties, making it effective for allergy relief.

4. Lemon (Citrus limon): Lemon oil may have antihistamine-like effects and can be refreshing when diffused.

5. Roman Chamomile (Chamaemelum nobile): Roman chamomile oil is known for its anti-inflammatory properties and can help soothe irritated nasal passages.

How to Use Essential Oils for Seasonal Allergies:

1. Aromatherapy Diffusion: Add a few drops of your chosen essential oil to an essential oil diffuser and inhale the aromatic mist. This method can help relieve symptoms and improve air quality indoors.

2. Steam Inhalation: Boil water, pour it into a bowl, and add a few drops of essential oil. Lean over the bowl with a towel covering your head and inhale the steam for relief.

3. Topical Application: Dilute essential oils with a carrier oil (such as coconut or almond oil) and apply the mixture to your chest, neck, and temples. This can provide localized relief.

4. Allergy-Relief Blends: Create custom blends by combining multiple essential oils known for their allergy-fighting properties. Experiment to find the blend that works best for you.

Safety Considerations:

- Always dilute essential oils before applying them to the skin.
- Conduct a patch test to check for any skin sensitivities or allergies.
- Consult with a healthcare professional, especially if you have allergies, asthma, or other underlying health conditions, before using essential oils.

Conclusion: Natural Allergy Relief

Essential oils offer a natural and holistic approach to managing seasonal allergies, providing relief from common symptoms without the side effects often associated with traditional medications. By incorporating the benefits of aromatherapy into your allergy management plan, you can enjoy the changing seasons with greater comfort and well-being. Experiment with different essential oils and application methods to find the natural relief that works best for you.

Exploring the World of Floral Essential Oils: Rose, Jasmine, and More

Introduction:

Floral essential oils, extracted from the delicate petals of flowers, are treasured for their enchanting aromas and a wide range of therapeutic benefits. Among these floral wonders, rose and jasmine essential oils stand out as some of the most prized and cherished essences in the world of aromatherapy. In this comprehensive text, we'll embark on a journey to explore the world of floral essential oils, their origins, therapeutic properties, and the fascinating ways they enhance our well-being and senses.

The Elegance of Floral Essential Oils:

Floral essential oils capture the essence and beauty of flowers, carrying their fragrance and therapeutic qualities in concentrated form. These oils are often used in perfumery, skincare, and aromatherapy for their captivating scents and holistic benefits.

Rose Essential Oil (Rosa damascena):

Origin: Rose essential oil is primarily extracted from the petals of the Damask rose, native to Bulgaria and Turkey.

Therapeutic Properties:

1. Emotional Healing: Rose oil is renowned for its ability to ease emotional distress, reduce stress, and alleviate symptoms of anxiety and depression.

2. Skin Nourishment: It is a luxurious oil for skincare, promoting a youthful complexion, reducing redness, and soothing irritation.

3. Aphrodisiac: Rose oil's romantic aroma is considered an aphrodisiac, enhancing sensuality and intimacy.

Jasmine Essential Oil (Jasminum grandiflorum):

Origin: Jasmine essential oil is typically extracted from the delicate blossoms of the jasmine plant, native to South Asia.

Therapeutic Properties:

1. Calming: Jasmine oil has a soothing and calming effect on the mind and body, reducing stress and anxiety.

2. Antidepressant: It is known for its mood-lifting properties and can help alleviate symptoms of depression.

3. Skin Rejuvenation: Jasmine oil is a popular ingredient in skincare products, promoting hydration and addressing dry or sensitive skin.

Other Floral Essential Oils:

1. Lavender (Lavandula angustifolia): While not solely a floral oil, lavender's sweet and herbaceous aroma makes it a beloved choice for relaxation and stress relief.

2. Chamomile (Matricaria chamomilla and Chamaemelum nobile): Chamomile essential oil, derived from the flowers of two different chamomile species, is renowned for its calming and soothing properties, making it ideal for promoting sleep and relaxation.

Practical Applications:

1. Aromatherapy: Add a few drops of floral essential oil to an essential oil diffuser to create a calming and uplifting atmosphere in your home.

2. Massage: Dilute floral oils with a carrier oil for a luxurious massage experience that promotes relaxation and emotional well-being.

3. Skincare: Incorporate floral essential oils into your skincare routine by adding a drop or two to your favorite moisturizer or facial oil.

4. Bath Soak: Enhance your bath with a few drops of floral oil for a spa-like experience that soothes the mind and body.

Safety Considerations:

- Always dilute essential oils before applying them to the skin, especially in sensitive areas.

- Conduct a patch test to check for any skin sensitivities or allergies.

- Consult with a healthcare professional if you are pregnant, nursing, or have any underlying health conditions before using essential oils.

Conclusion: Blooming Wellness with Florals

Floral essential oils, with their captivating scents and therapeutic properties, offer a sensory journey that promotes emotional well-being, relaxation, and skin health. Whether you're seeking solace in the delicate petals of rose and jasmine or exploring the calming embrace of lavender and chamomile, the world of floral essential oils invites you to embrace the beauty and holistic benefits of nature's most cherished blossoms. Incorporate these exquisite oils into your daily rituals, and let their fragrance and therapeutic properties enhance your well-being and elevate your senses.

Essential Oils for Spiritual Growth and Meditation

Introduction:

The use of essential oils for spiritual growth and meditation has been a practice for centuries, rooted in the belief that these aromatic essences can enhance mindfulness, deepen meditation, and promote a sense of inner peace. In this comprehensive text, we will explore the world of essential oils as powerful tools for spiritual development, delving into their origins, their impact on the mind and spirit, and practical ways to incorporate them into your meditation and spiritual practice.

The Ancient Connection:

Essential oils have played a significant role in various spiritual and religious traditions across cultures and centuries. From the use of frankincense and myrrh in ancient rituals to the sacred oils of Hinduism and Buddhism, aromatics have been recognized for their ability to elevate the spirit and create a bridge between the material and spiritual worlds.

Essential Oils and the Mind-Body Connection:

The therapeutic properties of essential oils extend beyond their pleasant scents; they interact with our senses, emotions, and even our brain chemistry. Here's how they influence the mind-body connection:

1. Aromatherapy: The inhalation of essential oil molecules triggers responses in the limbic system, which is responsible for emotions, memories, and mood.

2. Emotional Balance: Certain essential oils, such as lavender and frankincense, can help reduce stress, anxiety, and emotional turmoil, creating an ideal state for meditation and spiritual reflection.

3. Enhanced Focus: Essential oils like peppermint and rosemary can improve mental clarity and concentration, allowing for a more profound meditation experience.

Essential Oils for Spiritual Growth:

1. Frankincense (Boswellia serrata): Revered for its grounding and centering properties, frankincense is often used to deepen meditation and connect with one's higher self.

2. Myrrh (Commiphora myrrha): Myrrh is associated with inner peace and spiritual awareness, making it a valuable companion in meditation practices.

3. Sandalwood (Santalum album): Sandalwood's woody aroma is known for its calming and meditative qualities, helping to quiet the mind and enhance mindfulness.

4. Patchouli (Pogostemon cablin): Patchouli oil is believed to aid in releasing negative emotions and encouraging a sense of spiritual growth and self-acceptance.

Practical Applications:

1. Diffusion: Add a few drops of your chosen essential oil to an essential oil diffuser during meditation sessions to create a peaceful and spiritually supportive environment.

2. Anointing: Apply a diluted essential oil blend to your pulse points or the third eye chakra before meditation to enhance your connection to the spiritual realm.

3. Bathing: Incorporate essential oils into your bath ritual to relax the body and mind before engaging in spiritual practice.

4. Cleansing: Use essential oils as part of a cleansing and purification ritual, anointing objects or spaces with intention.

Safety Considerations:

- Always dilute essential oils before applying them to the skin, especially in sensitive areas.

- Conduct a patch test to check for any skin sensitivities or allergies.

- Use essential oils mindfully and sparingly during spiritual practices.

Essential oils can serve as valuable companions on your journey of spiritual growth and meditation. Their profound impact on the mind-body connection, emotions, and consciousness makes them powerful tools for enhancing mindfulness and deepening your spiritual practice. By incorporating the scents and energies of these sacred essences into your daily rituals, you can create a harmonious and spiritually enriching environment that supports your inner journey toward greater self-awareness and enlightenment.

Essential Oils for Sleep: A Natural Approach to Insomnia

Introduction:

Quality sleep is essential for overall health and well-being, yet many people struggle with insomnia and sleep-related issues. Essential oils, with their calming and soothing properties, offer a natural and holistic approach to improving sleep quality and overcoming insomnia. In this comprehensive text, we will explore the world of essential oils as a natural remedy for sleep problems, including their origins, benefits, practical application methods, and tips for creating a tranquil sleep environment.

Understanding Insomnia:

Insomnia is a common sleep disorder characterized by difficulty falling asleep, staying asleep, or experiencing restorative sleep. It can result in daytime fatigue, irritability, and a host of health issues.

Benefits of Essential Oils for Sleep:

1. Relaxation: Essential oils have calming and soothing properties that help relax the nervous system and prepare the body for sleep.

2. Stress Reduction: Aromatherapy with soothing oils can alleviate stress and anxiety, common contributors to insomnia.

3. Improved Sleep Quality: Essential oils can enhance the overall quality of sleep, leading to more restorative rest.

Popular Essential Oils for Sleep:

1. Lavender (Lavandula angustifolia): Lavender oil is renowned for its calming and soothing effects, making it a top choice for sleep support.

2. Chamomile (Matricaria chamomilla and Chamaemelum nobile): Chamomile essential oil has gentle, calming properties that promote relaxation and restful sleep.

3. Cedarwood (Cedrus atlantica): Cedarwood oil's earthy scent can induce a sense of tranquility and help with sleep onset.

4. Frankincense (Boswellia serrata): Frankincense is known for its grounding qualities and ability to ease stress, making it beneficial for sleep.

Practical Applications:

1. Aromatherapy Diffusion: Add a few drops of your chosen essential oil to an essential oil diffuser in your bedroom to create a calming and sleep-inducing atmosphere.

2. Topical Application: Dilute essential oils with a carrier oil (such as jojoba or coconut oil) and apply the mixture to your pulse points, neck, or the soles of your feet before bedtime.

3. Pillow Spray: Create a DIY pillow spray by mixing water and a few drops of essential oil in a spray bottle. Lightly spritz your pillow and bedding.

4. Bath Soak: Enjoy a relaxing bath before bedtime by adding a few drops of essential oil to your bathwater.

Creating a Tranquil Sleep Environment:

1. Dim the Lights: Use soft, dim lighting in your bedroom to signal to your body that it's time to wind down.

2. Reduce Noise: Minimize disruptive noises by using earplugs or a white noise machine.

3. Comfortable Bedding: Invest in a comfortable mattress and pillows that support your sleep ure.

4. Cool Temperature: Keep your bedroom cool, as a lower room temperature can promote better sleep.

5. Limit Screen Time: Avoid screens (phones, tablets, computers) before bedtime, as the blue light emitted can interfere with sleep.

Safety Considerations:

- Always dilute essential oils before applying them to the skin, especially in sensitive areas.
- Conduct a patch test to check for any skin sensitivities or allergies.
- Use essential oils mindfully and sparingly, as excessive use can have the opposite effect.

Conclusion: Sweet Dreams with Essential Oils

Essential oils offer a natural and soothing approach to improving sleep quality and managing insomnia. By incorporating the calming scents and therapeutic benefits of these precious essences into your bedtime routine and creating a tranquil sleep environment, you can embark on a journey toward restful and rejuvenating sleep. Embrace the power of aromatherapy as a gentle yet effective remedy for sleep-related issues, and let the comforting embrace of essential oils guide you to sweet dreams and a refreshed morning.

The Art of Perfumery: Crafting Fine Fragrances with Oils

Introduction:

Perfumery is a captivating art that has been cherished for centuries, with roots tracing back to ancient civilizations. The art of crafting fine fragrances involves blending essential oils, aromatic compounds, and other ingredients to create alluring scents that evoke emotions, memories, and experiences. In this comprehensive text, we will explore the world of perfumery, its rich history, the key components of fragrances, and the creative process behind crafting your own signature scent.

A Fragrant History:

Perfumery has a storied history, dating back to ancient Egypt, Mesopotamia, and the Indus Valley. Fragrance was considered a symbol of luxury, spirituality, and status, with perfumers using natural ingredients like flowers, herbs, and resins to create aromatic concoctions.

The Components of Fragrances:

1. Fragrance Oils: These are the heart of any perfume, and they provide the scent profile. Fragrance oils can be natural (essential oils) or synthetic (aromatic compounds).

2. Solvents: Solvents are used to dilute and stabilize fragrance oils. Common solvents include alcohol, jojoba oil, or fractionated coconut oil.

3. Fixatives: Fixatives help retain the scent of the perfume on the skin. Ingredients like benzoin, musk, and ambergris are traditional fixatives.

4. Modifiers: Modifiers are added to enhance or modify the fragrance. They can include ingredients like citral or aldehyde C14.

The Art of Perfume Blending:

Creating a perfume involves meticulously blending various fragrance oils, solvents, fixatives, and modifiers. Perfumers rely on their sensory perception, intuition, and creativity to craft harmonious scent compositions. The process typically involves three distinct notes:

1. Top Notes: These are the initial scents that are detected when the perfume is first applied. They are often light and refreshing, with ingredients like citrus, fruit, or herbs.

2. Middle Notes (Heart Notes): Middle notes emerge once the top notes have evaporated. They form the core of the fragrance and include floral and spice elements.

3. Base Notes: Base notes are the foundation of the perfume and are responsible for its longevity. They are often rich and woody, with ingredients like vanilla, musk, or amber.

Creating Your Signature Scent:

Crafting your own signature fragrance can be a deeply personal and creative endeavor. Here are some steps to get started:

1. Gather Materials: Acquire a range of essential oils, fragrance oils, and other perfumery ingredients.

2. Start with a Base: Choose a base note that resonates with you, as it will set the foundation for your fragrance.

3. Experiment and Blend: Begin blending different oils and modifiers, taking careful notes of each combination. Allow the blends to sit for a few days to mature and develop.

4. Refine and Adjust: Refine your blends by adjusting the ratios of ingredients until you achieve the desired scent.

5. Allow Maturation: Let your final blend mature for several weeks to fully develop its complexity and character.

6. Bottle and Enjoy: Once satisfied with your creation, bottle it in a dark, airtight container to preserve its aroma.

Safety Considerations:

- Some essential oils can be skin irritants or allergens. Perform a patch test before applying your fragrance to your skin.
- Be mindful of the concentration of fragrance oils in your blend, as too high a concentration can be overwhelming.

Conclusion: A Fragrant Journey

The art of perfumery is a sensory adventure that combines science, creativity, and an appreciation for the beauty of scent. Crafting your own fragrance allows you to express your individuality and create a scent that resonates with your unique personality.

Whether you're exploring perfumery as a hobby or a profession, the world of fine fragrances invites you to embark on a fragrant journey that captivates the senses and leaves a lasting impression.

Frankincense and Myrrh: Sacred Resins in Essential Oil Form

Introduction:

Frankincense and myrrh, two ancient resins with a rich history spanning thousands of years, have long held a revered place in spiritual, religious, and therapeutic practices. These sacred resins, once considered gifts fit for kings, have been transformed into essential oils, making their profound benefits and aromatic allure more accessible than ever. In this comprehensive text, we will delve into the origins, therapeutic properties, and versatile uses of frankincense and myrrh essential oils, uncovering the secrets of these sacred treasures.

Ancient Origins:

Frankincense and myrrh have been treasured since ancient times, with their roots dating back to the ancient civilizations of Egypt, Mesopotamia, and beyond. They were used in religious rituals, embalming, perfumery, and traditional medicine. These resins were considered precious commodities and were even presented as gifts to deities and rulers.

Frankincense Essential Oil (Boswellia spp.):

Origin: Frankincense essential oil is derived from the resin of various species of the Boswellia tree, native to regions like Oman, Yemen, and Somalia.

Therapeutic Properties:

1. Mood Elevation: Frankincense oil is renowned for its ability to induce feelings of calm, serenity, and spiritual connection.

2. Anti-Inflammatory: It has anti-inflammatory properties that can soothe joint pain and inflammation.

3. Skin Rejuvenation: Frankincense is used in skincare to promote a youthful complexion and reduce the appearance of blemishes and imperfections.

Myrrh Essential Oil (Commiphora spp.):

Origin: Myrrh essential oil is obtained from the resin of Commiphora species, primarily found in regions like Somalia and Ethiopia.

Therapeutic Properties:

1. Emotional Balance: Myrrh oil is known for its grounding and emotionally stabilizing effects, making it valuable for meditation and mindfulness.

2. Antiseptic: It possesses antiseptic properties and can be used for oral hygiene and wound care.

3. Skin Care: Myrrh is used to support healthy skin and address skin conditions.

Versatile Uses:

1. Aromatherapy: Both frankincense and myrrh essential oils are popular choices for diffusing during meditation, prayer, or yoga practices to enhance spiritual connection and relaxation.

2. Skincare: These oils can be added to your skincare routine to promote healthy, radiant skin. They are particularly beneficial for mature or blemish-prone skin.

3. Massage: Diluted in a carrier oil, frankincense and myrrh essential oils make excellent additions to massage blends, helping relax both the body and mind.

4. Oral Care: Myrrh essential oil can be diluted in water and used as a mouthwash to support oral health and hygiene.

5. Wound Care: Both oils have historically been used to cleanse and support the healing of wounds and skin irritations.

Safety Considerations:

- Always dilute essential oils before applying them to the skin.
- Conduct a patch test to check for any skin sensitivities or allergies.
- Consult with a healthcare professional, especially if you are pregnant, nursing, or have underlying health conditions.

Conclusion: Embracing Ancient Wisdom

Frankincense and myrrh essential oils carry the timeless wisdom of ancient civilizations and continue to provide a bridge between the past and the present. These sacred resins, now available in essential oil form, offer a range of physical, emotional, and spiritual benefits, making them valuable additions to modern wellness practices. By incorporating the enchanting scents and therapeutic properties of frankincense and myrrh into your daily rituals, you can connect with the wisdom of ages past and experience their profound effects on your well-being and spirituality.

The Role of Essential Oils in Ayurvedic Medicine

Introduction:

Ayurveda, the ancient system of natural medicine originating in India, has been enhancing health and well-being for over 5,000 years. At the heart of Ayurveda is the use of natural remedies, including essential oils, to balance the body, mind, and spirit. In this comprehensive text, we will explore the profound role of essential oils in Ayurvedic medicine, their connection to the doshas, and how they can be harnessed to promote holistic health and harmony.

The Essence of Ayurveda:

Ayurveda, often referred to as the "science of life," is built on the fundamental principle that individuals possess unique constitutional types, known as doshas. These doshas, named Vata, Pitta, and Kapha, represent the interplay of the five elements (earth, water, fire, air, and ether) within each person. Ayurvedic medicine seeks to maintain or restore balance within these doshas to achieve optimal health.

Essential Oils in Ayurveda:

Essential oils play a pivotal role in Ayurvedic healing due to their ability to address imbalances within the doshas. Each essential oil is classified according to its specific properties, which can either balance or aggravate the doshas. Here's a closer look at how essential oils align with the doshas:

1. Vata Dosha:

- Vata is characterized by qualities of air and ether, representing movement, creativity, and change.

- Essential oils that are warming, grounding, and calming are beneficial for balancing Vata.

- Examples: Lavender, Sandalwood, and Ginger.

2. Pitta Dosha:

- Pitta embodies qualities of fire and water, governing digestion, metabolism, and determination.

- Cooling and soothing essential oils help pacify Pitta dosha.

- Examples: Peppermint, Rose, and Coriander.

3. Kapha Dosha:

- Kapha is linked to earth and water elements, symbolizing stability, endurance, and nourishment.

- Essential oils with invigorating, uplifting, and stimulating properties can balance Kapha.

- Examples: Eucalyptus, Lemon, and Basil.

Practical Applications:

1. Abhyanga (Self-Massage): Ayurvedic self-massage with warm, dosha-balancing oils like sesame, coconut, or almond oil is a daily ritual that enhances circulation, relaxes the body, and promotes overall well-being.

2. Aromatherapy: Diffusing essential oils according to your dosha or imbalances can help create an environment conducive to balance and relaxation.

3. Herbal Combinations: Ayurvedic practitioners often combine essential oils with herbs to create custom blends for specific health concerns or imbalances.

4. Nasya (Nasal Administration): A few drops of dosha-specific oils are applied to the nasal passages to promote clarity, focus, and sinus health.

5. Holistic Healing: Essential oils are incorporated into Ayurvedic treatments like Panchakarma (detoxification) and Shirodhara (forehead oil flow) to support healing and rejuvenation.

Safety Considerations:

- Ayurvedic essential oil blends should be carefully chosen based on your dosha and the current state of balance or imbalance.

- Always dilute essential oils before applying them to the skin.

- It is advisable to consult with a qualified Ayurvedic practitioner for personalized recommendations.

Conclusion: Balancing Body, Mind, and Spirit

Essential oils are a cornerstone of Ayurvedic medicine, offering a natural and holistic approach to achieving balance within the doshas and promoting health on all levels. By understanding the unique qualities of each dosha and harnessing the therapeutic properties of essential oils, individuals can embark on a journey toward holistic well-being that encompasses not only physical health but also mental and spiritual harmony. Ayurveda invites us to explore the profound synergy between essential oils and the ancient wisdom of Ayurvedic healing, providing a path to balance, vitality, and enduring health.

How to Safely Use Essential Oils During Pregnancy

Introduction:

Pregnancy is a special and transformative time in a woman's life, often accompanied by a heightened awareness of health and well-being. Essential oils, with their therapeutic properties and pleasant aromas, can offer comfort and support during this journey. However, it's crucial to exercise caution and adhere to safety guidelines when using essential oils during pregnancy. In this comprehensive text, we will explore how to safely incorporate essential oils into your prenatal routine, potential benefits, and essential precautions to ensure a healthy and joyful pregnancy.

The Benefits of Essential Oils During Pregnancy:

1. Relaxation: Many essential oils have calming properties that can help reduce stress and anxiety, promoting emotional well-being during pregnancy.

2. Nausea Relief: Certain oils, such as ginger and peppermint, can alleviate nausea and morning sickness.

3. Skin Support: Essential oils like lavender and chamomile can help soothe skin irritations and reduce the appearance of stretch marks.

4. Better Sleep: Aromatherapy with relaxing oils can improve sleep quality, which is often disrupted during pregnancy.

Safety Guidelines for Using Essential Oils During Pregnancy:

1. Consult Your Healthcare Provider: Before using any essential oils during pregnancy, it's crucial to consult with your healthcare provider to ensure they are safe for your specific situation.

2. Dilution: Always dilute essential oils in a carrier oil (such as jojoba, coconut, or almond oil) before applying them to your skin. A general guideline is 1% to 2% dilution, which equates to 1 to 2 drops of essential oil per teaspoon of carrier oil.

3. Limited Application: Apply essential oil blends sparingly and only to specific areas of your body, avoiding sensitive areas, mucous membranes, and direct application on the abdomen or breasts.

4. Avoid Certain Oils: Some essential oils should be avoided during pregnancy due to their potential to stimulate uterine contractions or other adverse effects. These include but are not limited to:

- Clary sage
- Rosemary
- Juniper berry

- Cinnamon
- Thyme
- Oregano
- Pennyroyal

Safe Essential Oils for Pregnancy:

1. Lavender (Lavandula angustifolia): Calming and soothing, lavender is a versatile oil that can support relaxation and sleep.

2. Chamomile (Matricaria chamomilla): Chamomile's gentle properties make it suitable for soothing skin irritations and promoting relaxation.

3. Ginger (Zingiber officinale): Helpful for alleviating nausea and digestive discomfort.

4. Lemon (Citrus limon): A refreshing oil that can improve mood and provide a sense of energy and vitality.

Application Methods:

1. Aromatherapy: Diffusing essential oils in a well-ventilated room can provide emotional support and improve the atmosphere.

2. Massage: Diluted essential oils can be used in prenatal massages to ease muscle tension, improve circulation, and promote relaxation.

3. Baths: Adding a few drops of safe essential oils to a warm bath can be a luxurious way to unwind and alleviate stress.

Final Thoughts: Your Health Comes First

While essential oils can be a valuable addition to your prenatal wellness routine, it's crucial to prioritize your health and the well-being of your baby. Always consult your healthcare provider before using essential oils during pregnancy, and adhere to safety guidelines and dilution ratios. By approaching the use of essential oils with care and mindfulness, you can harness their therapeutic benefits and enjoy a healthier and more relaxed pregnancy journey.

Essential Oils for Hair Growth: Revitalize Your Locks

Introduction:

Healthy and vibrant hair is often seen as a symbol of beauty and vitality. If you're looking to enhance your hair's growth and overall condition, essential oils can be a natural and effective solution. In this comprehensive text, we will explore the world of essential oils for hair growth, their mechanisms of action, and how to incorporate them into your hair care routine to achieve luscious and revitalized locks.

Understanding Hair Growth:

Before delving into essential oils, it's essential to understand the basics of hair growth:

1. Anagen Phase: This is the active growth phase of the hair follicles, during which hair can grow up to 1 cm per month.

2. Catagen Phase: In this transitional phase, hair growth slows down as the follicle detaches from the blood supply.

3. Telogen Phase: The resting phase when hair is no longer growing and may eventually shed.

4. Exogen Phase: This is the natural shedding phase when old hairs are replaced by new ones.

How Essential Oils Promote Hair Growth:

Essential oils can influence hair growth through several mechanisms:

1. Improved Blood Circulation: Some essential oils, when massaged onto the scalp, can enhance blood flow to the hair follicles, promoting nutrient delivery and hair growth.

2. Strengthening Hair Follicles: Essential oils contain compounds that strengthen hair follicles, reducing breakage and hair loss.

3. Balancing Scalp Health: A healthy scalp is essential for hair growth. Essential oils with antifungal and antibacterial properties can maintain scalp health.

4. Reducing DHT: Dihydrotestosterone (DHT) is a hormone linked to hair loss. Some essential oils can inhibit DHT production.

Top Essential Oils for Hair Growth:

1. Lavender (Lavandula angustifolia): Lavender oil promotes hair growth by increasing blood circulation to the scalp and reducing stress, which can contribute to hair loss.

2. Rosemary (Rosmarinus officinalis): Rosemary oil strengthens hair follicles, improves hair thickness, and can help slow down hair loss.

3. Peppermint (Mentha piperita): Peppermint oil increases blood flow to the scalp, promoting hair growth and reducing hair loss.

4. Cedarwood (Cedrus atlantica): Cedarwood oil balances oil production in the scalp and can help reduce dandruff, creating a healthier environment for hair growth.

5. Jojoba (Simmondsia chinensis): Jojoba oil closely resembles the sebum produced by the scalp, making it an excellent moisturizer and hair growth enhancer.

Incorporating Essential Oils into Your Hair Care Routine:

1. Scalp Massage: Dilute a few drops of your chosen essential oil in a carrier oil like jojoba or coconut oil. Massage the mixture into your scalp for 5-10 minutes before shampooing.

2. Shampoo and Conditioner: Look for hair care products that contain essential oils or add a few drops of essential oil to your regular shampoo or conditioner.

3. Hair Masks: Create a nourishing hair mask by combining essential oils with yogurt, honey, or avocado. Apply to your hair and scalp for 30 minutes before washing.

4. Leave-In Treatments: Mix a few drops of essential oil with water in a spray bottle and spritz it onto your hair and scalp as a leave-in treatment.

Safety Considerations:

- Always dilute essential oils before applying them to the scalp or hair to prevent skin irritation.
- Perform a patch test to check for any allergic reactions or sensitivities.
- Consult with a dermatologist or healthcare provider if you have any underlying scalp conditions or hair loss concerns.

Conclusion: Unlocking the Potential of Essential Oils for Hair Growth

Essential oils offer a natural and holistic approach to promoting hair growth and maintaining healthy locks. By incorporating these oils into your hair care routine, you can enhance blood circulation to the scalp, strengthen hair follicles, and create a healthier environment for hair growth. Remember to exercise caution, use proper dilution, and consult with a healthcare provider if you have specific hair loss concerns. With consistent care and the power of essential oils, you can revitalize your locks and embrace the beauty of healthy, vibrant hair.

The Chemistry of Essential Oils: Terpenes, Alcohols, and More

Introduction:

Essential oils are prized for their captivating scents and therapeutic properties, but their magic lies in the intricate chemistry that makes them so versatile. These aromatic compounds are composed of a wide range of chemical constituents, each with its unique properties and benefits. In this comprehensive text, we will explore the fascinating chemistry of essential oils, focusing on some of the key chemical groups that give these oils their characteristic aroma and therapeutic effects.

The Building Blocks of Essential Oils: Chemical Constituents

1. Terpenes: Aromatic Hydrocarbons

Terpenes are the most abundant class of compounds in essential oils and are responsible for their distinct scents. They are composed of carbon and hydrogen atoms arranged in a specific pattern. Terpenes can be further categorized into monoterpenes and sesquiterpenes:

- Monoterpenes: These are composed of two isoprene units (a total of ten carbon atoms) and are found in oils like lemon (limonene) and lavender (linalool).

- Sesquiterpenes: These contain three isoprene units (a total of fifteen carbon atoms) and are present in oils like cedarwood (cedrol) and ginger (zingiberene).

2. Alcohols: Hydroxyl Groups

Alcohols are another essential oil component characterized by the presence of hydroxyl (-OH) groups. They contribute to the oils' antimicrobial and anti-inflammatory properties. Common alcohol constituents include:

- Linalool: Found in lavender and coriander oils, linalool has a calming and soothing effect.
- Geraniol: Present in rose and geranium oils, geraniol offers a sweet and floral aroma.
- Citronellol: Found in rose and geranium oils, citronellol has a fresh, rosy scent.

3. Ketones: C=O Functional Group

Ketones contain a carbonyl group (C=O) and are known for their powerful aroma and potential toxicity if used in excessive amounts. Notable ketones include:

- Camphor: Found in camphor oil, it has a cooling and penetrating scent.

- Menthone: Present in peppermint and spearmint oils, menthone provides a refreshing and invigorating aroma.

4. Esters: Ester Linkages

Esters are responsible for the fruity and sweet notes in essential oils. They are formed by the reaction of alcohols and acids. Common esters include:

- Linalyl acetate: Found in lavender and clary sage oils, it has a sweet and floral aroma.

- Geranyl acetate: Present in rose and geranium oils, geranyl acetate contributes to their fruity scent.

5. Phenols: Hydroxyl Group Attached to Benzene Ring

Phenols are characterized by the presence of a hydroxyl group (-OH) attached to a benzene ring. They have strong antimicrobial properties. Notable phenols include:

- Eugenol: Found in clove and cinnamon oils, eugenol has a spicy and warming scent.

- Thymol: Present in thyme and oregano oils, thymol has potent antibacterial properties.

Using Chemistry to Harness Essential Oil Benefits:

Understanding the chemistry of essential oils allows for targeted use and blending to achieve specific therapeutic effects:

- Balancing Blends: Combining oils with complementary chemical constituents can create balanced and effective blends. For example, mixing oils high in monoterpenes (like lemon) with oils high in sesquiterpenes (like cedarwood) can offer both uplifting and grounding effects.

- Safety: Knowing the chemical makeup of an oil can help assess its safety, as some constituents may be contraindicated for certain conditions or populations.

- Aroma Profiling: Recognizing the dominant chemical constituents in an oil can give insight into its aroma profile and potential uses. Oils high in alcohols (like linalool) tend to have a softer, floral scent, while oils high in phenols (like eugenol) have a spicier aroma.

Conclusion: The Art and Science of Essential Oils

The chemistry of essential oils is a blend of art and science, contributing to the diverse and beneficial properties these oils offer. By understanding the chemical constituents that make up essential oils, you can better appreciate their therapeutic potential and create customized blends that cater to your specific needs. Whether you're seeking relaxation, revitalization, or other wellness benefits, essential oils, with their complex chemistry, provide a holistic approach to improving your physical and emotional well-being.

Topical vs. Internal Use: When and How to Ingest Essential Oils

Introduction:

The use of essential oils has gained popularity for their diverse therapeutic benefits, including relaxation, immune support, and mood enhancement. Two common methods of using essential oils are topically (applied to the skin) and internally (ingested or consumed). However, understanding when and how to ingest essential oils safely is essential to ensure their effectiveness and avoid potential risks. In this comprehensive text, we will explore the differences between topical and internal use of essential oils, their benefits, precautions, and guidelines for safe application.

Topical Use of Essential Oils:

Topical application involves diluting essential oils in a carrier oil and applying them to the skin. Here are some key considerations for topical use:

Benefits:

1. Skin Health: Topical application can improve skin health by addressing issues such as acne, dryness, and inflammation.

2. Localized Relief: Essential oils can be applied directly to specific areas of the body to target pain, tension, or discomfort.

3. Aromatherapy: Topical application allows you to enjoy the aromatic benefits of essential oils throughout the day.

Precautions:

- Dilution: Essential oils should always be diluted in a carrier oil to prevent skin irritation. A common dilution ratio is 2-3 drops of essential oil per teaspoon of carrier oil.

- Patch Test: Before applying an essential oil blend to a larger area, perform a patch test on a small part of your skin to check for any allergic reactions or sensitivities.

- Sensitivity: Some individuals may have sensitive skin and may need to further dilute essential oils or use oils that are known to be gentle, like lavender or chamomile.

Internal Use of Essential Oils:

Internal use involves consuming essential oils by adding them to food, beverages, or capsules. Here are some considerations for internal use:

Benefits:

1. Digestive Support: Some essential oils can support digestion and help alleviate symptoms like bloating and indigestion.

2. Flavor Enhancement: Essential oils can add unique and intense flavors to dishes and beverages.

3. Convenience: Internal use can be a convenient way to incorporate essential oils into your daily routine.

Precautions:

- Quality Matters: Only use high-quality, therapeutic-grade essential oils that are labeled for internal use. Not all essential oils are safe to ingest.

- Moderation: Essential oils are potent, and a little goes a long way. Start with a single drop and gradually increase as needed and under the advisement of a reputable provider/manufacturer.

- Dilution: When using essential oils in cooking, dilute them by mixing them with a carrier oil, honey, or another medium to disperse the oil evenly.

- Consult a Professional: If you have specific health concerns or conditions, consult a qualified aromatherapist, herbalist, or healthcare provider before ingesting essential oils.

Safe Ways to Ingest Essential Oils:

1. Culinary Use: Add a drop or less of food-grade essential oils to recipes, beverages, or dishes for flavor enhancement. Common culinary oils include lemon, peppermint, and lavender.

2. Capsules: Some individuals prefer encapsulating essential oils in vegetable capsules for easy ingestion. This method allows for precise dosing.

3. Beverages: Stirring a drop of essential oil into a glass of water, tea, or smoothie can provide flavor and potential health benefits.

Conclusion: Safety and Personalization

The choice between topical and internal use of essential oils depends on your specific needs and preferences. Both methods can provide therapeutic benefits when used safely and thoughtfully. Remember that essential oils are potent substances, so always prioritize safety by diluting them, performing patch tests, and using high-quality oils. When in doubt, seek guidance from a qualified aromatherapist or healthcare professional to ensure you're making the most of these aromatic treasures while safeguarding your well-being.

Essential Oils for Mental Clarity and Focus

Introduction:

In today's fast-paced world, maintaining mental clarity and focus is crucial for productivity, creativity, and overall well-being. Essential oils, with their natural aromas and therapeutic properties, can be powerful allies in enhancing mental clarity and concentration. In this comprehensive text, we will explore the world of essential oils for mental clarity and focus, their mechanisms of action, and practical ways to incorporate them into your daily routine to boost cognitive performance.

The Science of Aromatherapy:

Aromatherapy, the practice of using essential oils to improve psychological and physical well-being, can positively impact mental clarity and focus through several mechanisms:

1. Olfactory System Stimulation: The olfactory system is closely linked to the brain's limbic system, which plays a key role in emotions, memory, and learning. Inhaling essential oils can stimulate the limbic system, influencing mood, memory, and cognitive function.

2. Stress Reduction: Many essential oils have calming and stress-reducing properties, which can help clear mental clutter and improve focus by reducing anxiety and tension.

3. Increased Blood Flow: Some essential oils, when inhaled, can increase blood flow to the brain, supplying it with more oxygen and nutrients, resulting in improved cognitive function.

Top Essential Oils for Mental Clarity and Focus:

1. Peppermint (Mentha piperita): Peppermint oil is renowned for its invigorating and stimulating aroma. It can improve alertness, concentration, and mental clarity.

2. Rosemary (Rosmarinus officinalis): Rosemary oil is a memory-enhancing oil that can help boost cognitive function, making it an excellent choice for studying and work tasks.

3. Lemon (Citrus limon): The fresh and uplifting scent of lemon oil can improve mood, increase alertness, and enhance mental clarity.

4. Lavender (Lavandula angustifolia): While commonly known for its calming properties, lavender oil can also promote mental clarity and focus by reducing stress and anxiety.

5. Eucalyptus (Eucalyptus globulus): Eucalyptus oil has a refreshing and invigorating scent that can help clear mental fog and improve concentration.

Practical Applications:

1. Diffusion: The most common way to enjoy the benefits of essential oils for mental clarity is through diffusion. Use an essential oil diffuser to disperse the aroma into your workspace or home.

2. Inhalation: Carry a small bottle of your chosen essential oil and inhale it directly from the bottle or apply a drop to a tissue or cotton ball to sniff throughout the day.

3. Topical Application: Dilute essential oils in a carrier oil (e.g., jojoba, coconut) and apply a small amount to your temples, wrists, or the back of your neck for a quick mental boost.

4. Aromatherapy Jewelry: Consider wearing aromatherapy jewelry, such as diffuser necklaces or bracelets, that allows you to carry the scent of essential oils with you wherever you go.

Safety Considerations:

- Always dilute essential oils before applying them to the skin, especially for topical use.

- Perform a patch test to check for any skin sensitivities or allergies.

- Use essential oils in moderation; a little goes a long way.

Conclusion: Unlocking Mental Clarity and Focus

Essential oils offer a natural and aromatic approach to achieving mental clarity and sharpening your focus. By incorporating these oils into your daily routine through diffusion, inhalation, or topical application, you can harness their power to reduce stress, increase alertness, and enhance cognitive performance. Remember to prioritize safety by using high-quality oils, proper dilution, and performing patch tests when necessary. With the delightful scents and therapeutic benefits of essential oils, you can elevate your mental clarity and focus, making each day more productive and fulfilling.

Essential Oils in History: From Cleopatra to the Renaissance

Introduction:

The use of essential oils spans millennia, with a rich history that weaves through ancient civilizations, influential figures, and diverse cultures. From the time of Cleopatra in ancient Egypt to the Renaissance period in Europe, essential oils have played a pivotal role in various aspects of life, including beauty, medicine, spirituality, and trade. In this comprehensive text, we will embark on a journey through history to explore the fascinating role of essential oils in different civilizations and their enduring legacy in the modern world.

Ancient Egypt: Perfumes and Healing Elixirs

1. Cleopatra's Beauty Regimen: The legendary Queen Cleopatra of Egypt is renowned for her beauty, and essential oils played a significant role in her daily regimen. She favored fragrant oils such as rose and lavender, using them in perfumes, bath oils, and skin treatments.

2. Healing Arts: In ancient Egypt, essential oils were used not only for their aromatic qualities but also for their medicinal properties. Egyptians infused oils with herbs and resins to create healing elixirs and embalming balms.

Ancient Greece and Rome: The Birth of Aromatherapy

1. Hippocrates and Dioscorides: Hippocrates, the father of medicine, and Dioscorides, the Greek physician and herbalist, wrote extensively on the therapeutic benefits of aromatic plants. They laid the foundation for what we now know as aromatherapy.

2. Roman Baths: Romans valued the use of essential oils in their elaborate bathhouses. Oils such as frankincense and myrrh were added to bathwater for their soothing and rejuvenating effects.

The Middle Ages: Essential Oils and Alchemy

1. Monastic Gardens: In medieval Europe, monasteries maintained gardens where monks cultivated aromatic herbs and plants for medicinal purposes. Essential oils were used in herbal remedies and tinctures.

2. Alchemy: During the Middle Ages, alchemists sought to transform base metals into gold and discovered the distillation process, a critical technique for extracting essential oils.

The Renaissance: Aromatic Renaissance

1. The Medicis and Catherine de' Medici: The influential Medici family of Florence, Italy, had a deep appreciation for fragrances. Catherine de'

Medici, as the Queen of France, introduced perfume to the French court, popularizing the use of essential oils in Europe.

2. Leonardo da Vinci: The Renaissance polymath Leonardo da Vinci documented the distillation process for essential oils in his notebooks, contributing to the understanding of their extraction.

Modern Revival: Rediscovering Aromatherapy

1. Renewed Interest: Aromatherapy experienced a resurgence in the 20th century, thanks to the pioneering work of figures like René-Maurice Gattefossé and Jean Valnet. Gattefossé's accidental discovery of lavender's healing properties led to the term "aromatherapy."

2. Scientific Validation: Modern research has confirmed many of the historical uses of essential oils. They are now used in various fields, including holistic health, spa and wellness, and even clinical settings.

Conclusion: The Timeless Elegance of Essential Oils

The history of essential oils is a testament to their enduring allure and practicality. From ancient Egypt to the Renaissance and beyond, these aromatic wonders have transcended time and continue to enrich our lives today. Whether used for beauty, medicine, or simply to elevate the senses, essential oils remain a source of fascination and inspiration, connecting us to the wisdom of our ancestors and the timeless beauty of nature's fragrant treasures.

The Benefits of Eucalyptus Oil for Respiratory Health

Introduction:

Eucalyptus oil, derived from the leaves of the eucalyptus tree (Eucalyptus globulus), has a long history of use for its therapeutic properties, particularly in supporting respiratory health. Its refreshing aroma and natural compounds make it a valuable tool for alleviating various respiratory issues. In this comprehensive text, we will explore the numerous benefits of eucalyptus oil for respiratory health, including its mechanisms of action, practical applications, and precautions.

Eucalyptus Oil's Respiratory Benefits:

1. Decongestant: Eucalyptus oil contains compounds like cineole, which have a decongestant effect on the respiratory system. Inhaling its vapor can help clear blocked nasal passages and ease breathing.

2. Expectorant: Eucalyptus oil can promote the loosening and expulsion of mucus from the airways, making it effective for relieving coughs and congestion.

3. Anti-Inflammatory: The anti-inflammatory properties of eucalyptus oil can help reduce inflammation in the respiratory tract, providing relief from conditions like bronchitis and asthma.

4. Antimicrobial: Eucalyptus oil exhibits antimicrobial properties that can combat respiratory infections caused by bacteria and viruses.

Practical Applications:

1. Steam Inhalation: Boil water, remove it from heat, and add a few drops of eucalyptus oil to create a steam inhalation. Cover your head with a towel, lean over the bowl, and inhale the steam deeply for 5-10 minutes to clear congestion.

2. Diffusion: Use an essential oil diffuser to disperse eucalyptus oil vapor into the air. This can help maintain a healthy respiratory environment in your living space.

3. Topical Application: Dilute eucalyptus oil with a carrier oil (e.g., coconut or olive oil) and apply it to your chest and throat. This can provide localized relief for respiratory discomfort.

4. Massage Oil: Mix eucalyptus oil with a carrier oil and use it for a soothing chest and back massage to relieve congestion and promote relaxation.

Precautions:

- Eucalyptus oil is potent and should be used in moderation. A few drops are usually sufficient.

- Do not ingest eucalyptus oil. It should only be used for topical and aromatic purposes.

- Perform a patch test to check for any skin sensitivities or allergies before applying it topically.

- Avoid using eucalyptus oil around young children or pets, as it can be toxic if ingested.

Conclusion: Embracing the Respiratory Benefits of Eucalyptus Oil

Eucalyptus oil stands as a versatile and natural remedy for maintaining respiratory health. Its decongestant, expectorant, anti-inflammatory, and antimicrobial properties make it a valuable addition to your wellness toolkit. Whether inhaled through steam, diffused in the air, or applied topically with care, eucalyptus oil can provide relief from respiratory discomfort and promote easier breathing. As with any essential oil, it's important to use eucalyptus oil thoughtfully and in accordance with safety guidelines to enjoy its full benefits for respiratory well-being.

Essential Oils for Weight Management: Suppressing Cravings

Introduction:

Weight management is a journey that involves various aspects of lifestyle, including diet, exercise, and mental well-being. Essential oils, with their natural aromas and therapeutic properties, can be valuable allies in your quest to control cravings and maintain a healthy weight. In this comprehensive text, we will explore the role of essential oils in suppressing cravings, their mechanisms of action, and practical ways to incorporate them into your wellness routine to support your weight management goals.

Cravings and Weight Management: The Challenge

Cravings, often for unhealthy and high-calorie foods, can be a significant hurdle in weight management. They are influenced by factors such as stress, emotions, hormonal fluctuations, and even environmental cues. Essential oils can provide a natural and holistic approach to addressing these triggers and promoting better control over cravings.

How Essential Oils Suppress Cravings:

1. Aromatherapy: Aromatherapy, the practice of inhaling the aroma of essential oils, can influence the brain's limbic system, which plays a role

in emotions, mood, and appetite control. Certain essential oils can promote feelings of satiety and reduce the desire for unhealthy foods.

2. Emotional Support: Many essential oils have mood-enhancing properties that can help combat emotional eating. By reducing stress, anxiety, and emotional triggers, essential oils can indirectly assist in managing cravings.

Top Essential Oils for Craving Control:

1. Peppermint (Mentha piperita): Peppermint oil is known for its invigorating aroma, which can reduce appetite and food cravings. Inhaling its scent can provide a sense of fullness and satisfaction.

2. Grapefruit (Citrus paradisi): Grapefruit oil has a bright and uplifting scent that can help curb sugar cravings. It may also support metabolism and fat breakdown.

3. Bergamot (Citrus bergamia): Bergamot oil has mood-enhancing properties and can reduce stress-related eating. It can uplift your mood and promote a sense of well-being.

4. Cinnamon (Cinnamomum verum): Cinnamon oil has a sweet and spicy aroma that can help regulate blood sugar levels, reducing cravings for sugary treats.

Practical Applications:

1. Aromatherapy Inhalation: Inhale the aroma directly from the bottle, add a few drops to a tissue or cotton ball, or use an essential oil diffuser to disperse the scent into your living space.

2. Topical Application: Dilute essential oils in a carrier oil (e.g., coconut or almond oil) and apply them to pulse points like wrists, temples, and the back of the neck.

3. Scented Jewelry: Consider wearing aromatherapy jewelry, such as diffuser necklaces or bracelets, to carry the craving-suppressing scent with you throughout the day.

4. Custom Blends: Create your own essential oil blends by combining oils that target different aspects of cravings, such as emotional triggers and appetite control.

Safety Considerations:

- Always dilute essential oils before applying them to the skin, especially for topical use.
- Perform a patch test to check for any skin sensitivities or allergies before applying essential oils.

- If you have underlying medical conditions or are pregnant or nursing, consult with a healthcare provider before using essential oils for weight management.

Conclusion: A Natural Approach to Craving Control

Essential oils offer a natural and aromatic solution to the challenge of cravings in your weight management journey. By incorporating these oils into your daily routine through inhalation, topical application, or the use of aromatherapy jewelry, you can harness their power to reduce appetite, enhance mood, and promote better control over food cravings. Remember that essential oils are a complementary approach and should be part of a holistic lifestyle that includes a balanced diet and regular exercise. With thoughtful use and a commitment to your well-being, essential oils can be valuable tools in supporting your weight management goals.

The Energetics of Essential Oils: Matching Scents to Mood

Introduction:

The world of essential oils extends beyond their pleasant aromas and therapeutic benefits; it delves into the realm of energy and emotion. The concept of the energetics of essential oils acknowledges that each oil carries a unique vibrational frequency that can influence our emotional and energetic states. In this comprehensive text, we will explore the fascinating world of essential oil energetics, how certain scents align with different moods, and practical ways to use them to enhance your well-being.

Understanding Essential Oil Energetics:

1. Vibrational Frequencies: Everything in the universe, including essential oils, emits a vibrational frequency. These frequencies can interact with our own energetic systems, impacting our emotions and moods.

2. Subtle Energy Systems: Many cultures, including Traditional Chinese Medicine and Ayurveda, recognize the existence of subtle energy systems in the body. Essential oils can influence these systems, promoting balance and harmony.

Matching Scents to Mood:

1. Calm and Relaxation: Lavender (Lavandula angustifolia): Lavender oil emits a calming and soothing energy, making it ideal for promoting relaxation and reducing stress.

2. Uplifting and Joyful: Sweet Orange (Citrus sinensis): Sweet orange oil exudes a bright and cheerful energy, lifting your spirits and promoting a positive mood.

3. Grounding and Centering: Patchouli (Pogostemon cablin): Patchouli oil carries an earthy and grounding energy that can help you feel centered and connected to the present moment.

4. Balancing and Harmonizing: Rose (Rosa damascena): Rose oil's gentle and harmonious energy can balance the heart chakra, promoting feelings of love and compassion.

5. Energizing and Invigorating: Peppermint (Mentha piperita): Peppermint oil's vibrant and invigorating energy can boost alertness and mental clarity.

Practical Applications:

1. Aromatherapy: Inhale the aroma directly from the bottle or use an essential oil diffuser to disperse the scent into your living space. Select oils that match your desired mood.

2. Topical Application: Dilute essential oils in a carrier oil and apply them to pulse points, such as wrists, temples, and the back of the neck, to infuse your energy with the oil's vibrational frequency.

3. Chakra Balancing: Explore chakra-based aromatherapy by using oils that align with specific energy centers to promote balance and alignment.

4. Meditation and Yoga: Incorporate essential oils into your meditation or yoga practice to enhance the energetic and emotional aspects of these practices.

Safety Considerations:

- Always dilute essential oils before applying them to the skin, especially for topical use.
- Perform a patch test to check for any skin sensitivities or allergies before applying essential oils.
- Use essential oils mindfully and in accordance with your personal preferences and sensitivities.

Conclusion: Elevating Well-Being Through Essential Oil Energetics

The energetics of essential oils provide a unique perspective on their power to influence our emotional and energetic states. By understanding the vibrational frequencies of different oils and matching them to your mood or intention, you can harness their energy to enhance your well-being. Whether you seek calm and relaxation, uplifting joy, or grounding and balance, essential oils offer a holistic and aromatic approach to aligning your energies and emotions with your desired state of being. Embrace the magic of essential oil energetics and allow their subtle energies to elevate your daily life.

Lavender Essential Oil: The Swiss Army Knife of Oils

Introduction:

Lavender essential oil, extracted from the lavender plant (Lavandula angustifolia), is often referred to as the "Swiss Army Knife" of essential oils due to its versatility and wide range of therapeutic properties. With a history dating back thousands of years, lavender oil has earned its place as one of the most popular and beloved essential oils. In this comprehensive text, we will explore the remarkable qualities of lavender essential oil and its many practical uses in aromatherapy, personal care, and wellness.

The Lavender Plant: A Timeless Treasure

Lavender, with its fragrant purple blooms and soothing aroma, has been cherished for centuries for its numerous benefits. Here are some of the key properties that make lavender essential oil a versatile essential oil:

1. Calming and Relaxing: Lavender oil is renowned for its calming and stress-relieving properties. Its scent can promote relaxation, reduce anxiety, and improve sleep quality.

2. Anti-Inflammatory: Lavender oil has anti-inflammatory properties that can soothe skin irritations, insect bites, and minor burns.

3. Antiseptic: It possesses natural antiseptic qualities, making it useful for cleaning wounds and promoting the healing of minor cuts and scrapes.

4. Pain Relief: Lavender oil can help alleviate headaches, muscle aches, and joint pain when applied topically or used in massage.

5. Skin Care: Lavender oil is gentle on the skin and can be used to improve the appearance of acne, scars, and blemishes.

Practical Uses of Lavender Essential Oil:

1. Aromatherapy: Diffuse lavender oil in your home or workplace to create a calming and relaxing atmosphere. It's especially beneficial before bedtime to promote restful sleep.

2. Topical Application: Dilute lavender oil with a carrier oil (e.g., coconut or jojoba oil) and apply it to the skin for soothing relief from minor skin irritations or to promote relaxation.

3. Bath Time: Add a few drops of lavender oil to your bathwater for a luxurious and calming spa-like experience.

4. Massage: Incorporate lavender oil into massage oil blends to relax muscles, reduce tension, and improve overall well-being.

5. Personal Care: Enhance your beauty and personal care routine by adding a drop of lavender oil to your moisturizer, shampoo, or body wash.

6. First Aid: Keep a small bottle of lavender oil in your first-aid kit to address minor burns, cuts, and insect bites.

Safety Considerations:

- Lavender oil is generally considered safe for most individuals when used properly, but it's advisable to perform a patch test before applying it to the skin.

- Pregnant and nursing women, as well as individuals with specific medical conditions or sensitivities, should consult a healthcare professional before using lavender oil.

Conclusion: Lavender Essential Oil, Your Versatile Companion

Lavender essential oil is a true multitasker, offering a wide range of benefits for your physical, emotional, and mental well-being. Whether you seek relaxation, relief from minor ailments, or a natural addition to your beauty routine, lavender oil has you covered. Its timeless and versatile nature makes it a must-have in every essential oil collection. Embrace the Swiss Army Knife of essential oils and allow lavender to enrich your life with its soothing and therapeutic qualities.

Aromatherapy in Hospitals: Complementary Healing Practices

Introduction:

Aromatherapy, the use of essential oils derived from plants for therapeutic purposes, has gained recognition and acceptance in healthcare settings, including hospitals, as a complementary healing practice. The soothing and healing properties of essential oils have found their place alongside conventional medical treatments, offering patients a holistic approach to wellness. In this comprehensive text, we will explore the role of aromatherapy in hospitals, its benefits, practical applications, and the growing acceptance of this complementary healing modality in healthcare.

Aromatherapy in Healthcare: A Brief Overview

Aromatherapy has a rich history dating back thousands of years, with roots in various cultures and healing traditions. In recent years, its integration into healthcare settings, particularly hospitals, has gained momentum. Here's an overview of its role:

1. Complementary Healing: Aromatherapy is used alongside conventional medical treatments to enhance the overall well-being of patients. It does not replace medical care but complements it.

2. Patient-Centered Care: Aromatherapy recognizes the importance of addressing not just physical symptoms but also the emotional and psychological needs of patients.

3. Essential Oils: High-quality essential oils are selected based on their therapeutic properties and are administered through inhalation, topical application, or, in some cases, ingestion (under the guidance of a trained practitioner).

Benefits of Aromatherapy in Hospitals:

1. Stress Reduction: Aromatherapy can reduce anxiety and stress levels among patients and healthcare professionals, promoting a calming and soothing atmosphere.

2. Pain Management: Certain essential oils have analgesic properties and can assist in pain management, providing relief from discomfort.

3. Improved Sleep: Aromatherapy can help patients improve the quality of their sleep, which is vital for healing and recovery.

4. Emotional Support: Essential oils can positively influence mood, providing emotional support to patients experiencing anxiety, depression, or grief.

5. Nausea Relief: Aromatherapy can help alleviate nausea and vomiting associated with medical treatments, such as chemotherapy.

Practical Applications:

1. Diffusion: Essential oil diffusers are used to disperse the aroma throughout patient rooms or waiting areas.

2. Topical Application: Diluted essential oils are applied to the skin through massage, compresses, or lotion to address specific issues.

3. Inhalation: Patients may inhale essential oils through steam inhalation, personal inhalers, or simply by sniffing from a tissue.

4. Personalized Blends: Trained aromatherapists can create customized essential oil blends tailored to individual patient needs.

Growing Acceptance in Healthcare:

1. Clinical Studies: A growing body of clinical research supports the effectiveness of aromatherapy in healthcare settings, prompting its integration into patient care plans.

2. Holistic Care: Hospitals are increasingly adopting holistic approaches to patient care, recognizing the interconnectedness of physical, emotional, and psychological well-being.

3. Patient Satisfaction: Aromatherapy contributes to improved patient satisfaction scores by providing a more positive and comfortable experience during hospital stays.

Safety Considerations:

- It's essential to use high-quality, therapeutic-grade essential oils.

- Aromatherapy should be administered by trained and certified practitioners to ensure safe and effective use.

Conclusion: Aromatherapy Enhancing Healthcare

Aromatherapy in hospitals is a testament to the evolving landscape of healthcare, where complementary and holistic practices are becoming integral to patient-centered care. As essential oils continue to demonstrate their therapeutic benefits, their role in reducing stress, managing pain, and providing emotional support cannot be understated. Hospitals and healthcare institutions are recognizing the value of aromatherapy as a holistic approach to healing, allowing patients to experience a greater sense of well-being during their healthcare journey. With its growing acceptance, aromatherapy is enhancing the overall quality of healthcare and offering patients a more comprehensive healing experience.

Essential Oils for Digestive Health: Alleviating Tummy Troubles

Introduction:

Digestive discomfort is a common concern that can disrupt daily life. Whether it's indigestion, bloating, or an upset stomach, essential oils offer a natural and effective way to support digestive health. In this comprehensive text, we will explore how essential oils can alleviate tummy troubles, their mechanisms of action, and practical ways to incorporate them into your wellness routine to promote digestive well-being.

Understanding Digestive Discomfort:

Digestive issues can arise from various factors, including poor dietary choices, stress, food sensitivities, and more. Essential oils can help address these concerns by providing relief from symptoms and promoting overall digestive health.

How Essential Oils Support Digestive Health:

1. Anti-Spasmodic: Some essential oils have anti-spasmodic properties, which means they can help relax the muscles of the digestive tract, reducing cramps and spasms.

2. Carminative: Carminative essential oils can help alleviate gas and bloating by aiding in the expulsion of excess gas from the digestive system.

3. Anti-Inflammatory: Essential oils with anti-inflammatory properties can reduce inflammation in the digestive tract, providing relief from conditions like gastritis or irritable bowel syndrome (IBS).

Top Essential Oils for Digestive Health:

1. Peppermint (Mentha piperita): Peppermint oil is known for its ability to relieve indigestion, bloating, and gas. It can also help relax the muscles of the gastrointestinal tract.

2. Ginger (Zingiber officinale): Ginger oil can alleviate nausea, promote healthy digestion, and reduce inflammation in the digestive system.

3. Lemon (Citrus limon): Lemon oil supports healthy liver function and can aid in detoxifying the digestive system.

4. Lavender (Lavandula angustifolia): Lavender oil's calming properties can help reduce stress-related digestive issues.

5. Fennel (Foeniculum vulgare): Fennel oil is a powerful carminative that can help relieve gas, bloating, and digestive discomfort.

Practical Applications:

1. Aromatherapy: Diffuse essential oils in your home to create a soothing environment that promotes relaxation and healthy digestion.

2. Topical Application: Dilute essential oils in a carrier oil and massage the blend onto your abdomen in a clockwise motion to support digestion.

3. Ingestion (with caution): Some essential oils can be ingested when properly diluted and under the guidance of a trained practitioner. Ensure you are using oils that are safe for consumption.

4. Tea or Water: Add a drop of food-grade essential oil to a warm cup of herbal tea or water for a gentle digestive boost.

Safety Considerations:

- Always dilute essential oils before applying them to the skin or ingesting them, and use them in moderation.
- Consult a healthcare professional before using essential oils for digestive issues, especially if you have underlying medical conditions or are pregnant or nursing.

Conclusion: Nurturing Digestive Wellness Naturally

Essential oils offer a holistic and natural approach to promoting digestive health and alleviating tummy troubles. By harnessing the anti-spasmodic, carminative, and anti-inflammatory properties of select oils, you can address common digestive discomforts and enhance overall well-being. Whether you choose to inhale the soothing aroma, apply oils topically, or use them in your favorite herbal tea, essential oils provide a gentle and effective way to nurture digestive wellness and keep tummy troubles at bay. Remember to use essential oils mindfully and consult with a healthcare professional for personalized guidance on addressing digestive issues.

The Role of Essential Oils in Yoga and Mindfulness

Introduction:

Yoga and mindfulness practices have long been celebrated for their profound effects on physical, mental, and emotional well-being. Essential oils, with their aromatic and therapeutic qualities, can enhance these practices by creating a sensory experience that deepens relaxation, focus, and self-awareness. In this comprehensive text, we will explore the harmonious relationship between essential oils, yoga, and mindfulness, and how they can elevate your practice and enrich your daily life.

Yoga and Mindfulness: A Holistic Approach to Well-Being

Yoga and mindfulness practices are grounded in the belief that physical health is intertwined with mental and emotional balance. Here's a brief overview of their core principles:

1. Yoga: Yoga is a holistic discipline that combines physical ures (asanas), breath control (pranayama), and meditation to promote physical strength, flexibility, mental clarity, and spiritual growth.

2. Mindfulness: Mindfulness involves being fully present in the moment, observing thoughts and emotions without judgment. It is practiced through meditation and mindfulness exercises to cultivate self-awareness and reduce stress.

The Synergy of Essential Oils:

Essential oils offer a complementary approach to yoga and mindfulness, enhancing the depth and effectiveness of these practices. Here's how they contribute:

1. Aromatherapy: The inhalation of essential oils during yoga and mindfulness sessions can influence the limbic system, the brain's emotional center. This can evoke feelings of relaxation, clarity, and focus.

2. Emotional Support: Certain essential oils have mood-balancing properties that can help reduce stress and anxiety, allowing for a more profound meditative experience.

3. Physical Comfort: Essential oils can soothe muscles and joints, enhancing the physical aspects of yoga. They can also promote deeper relaxation during savasana (corpse pose).

Choosing Essential Oils for Yoga and Mindfulness:

1. Lavender (Lavandula angustifolia): Lavender oil promotes relaxation and reduces stress, making it ideal for restorative yoga and mindfulness meditation.

2. Frankincense (Boswellia carterii): Frankincense oil enhances focus and deepens meditation. It has a grounding aroma that supports spiritual practices.

3. Peppermint (Mentha piperita): Peppermint oil can invigorate the mind and body, making it suitable for dynamic yoga styles and energizing mindfulness practices.

4. Bergamot (Citrus bergamia): Bergamot oil has mood-lifting properties and is excellent for balancing emotions during mindfulness and meditation.

5. Sandalwood (Santalum album): Sandalwood oil is deeply grounding and enhances inner peace and spiritual connection.

Practical Applications:

1. Diffusion: Use an essential oil diffuser in your yoga or meditation space to create an aromatic atmosphere that enhances your practice.

2. Topical Application: Dilute essential oils in a carrier oil and apply them to pulse points or the soles of your feet before practice.

3. Aromatic Mists: Create an aromatic mist by combining essential oils with water in a spray bottle. Mist your yoga mat or meditation cushion for an immersive experience.

4. DIY Blends: Experiment with creating your own essential oil blends that resonate with your intention for each practice.

Safety Considerations:

- Ensure that you are using high-quality, pure essential oils free from synthetic additives.
- Dilute essential oils appropriately when applying them to the skin, especially before yoga, to prevent skin sensitivities.

Conclusion: Elevating Your Practice with Essential Oils

Essential oils are a harmonious companion to yoga and mindfulness, enhancing the physical, mental, and emotional aspects of these practices. By incorporating aromatherapy into your routine, you can create a sensory experience that deepens relaxation, focus, and self-awareness. Whether you seek to calm your mind, energize your body, or deepen your spiritual connection, essential oils offer a versatile and natural way to elevate your practice and enrich your daily life. Embrace the synergy of essential oils, yoga, and mindfulness to nurture your holistic well-being and cultivate a sense of inner harmony.

Safety Precautions When Using Essential Oils with Children

Introduction:

The use of essential oils in aromatherapy and holistic wellness has become increasingly popular, but when it comes to using essential oils with children, extra care and caution are essential. Children's developing bodies and sensitive skin require a different approach to ensure their safety and well-being. In this comprehensive text, we will explore important safety precautions and guidelines for using essential oils with children, helping you make informed choices that support their health and comfort.

Understanding Essential Oils and Children:

1. Age Matters: Children of different ages have varying levels of sensitivity to essential oils. It's crucial to consider a child's age when choosing which oils to use and how to dilute them.

2. Skin Sensitivity: Children typically have more delicate and sensitive skin than adults, making them more prone to skin reactions from undiluted essential oils.

3. Physiological Differences: Children's bodies process substances differently than adults. Their developing organs, especially the liver

and kidneys, may not efficiently metabolize certain compounds found in essential oils.

Safety Precautions for Using Essential Oils with Children:

1. Age Appropriateness: Essential oils should not be used on infants under three months of age. For older children, research age-appropriate essential oils and their recommended dilutions.

2. Dilution: Always dilute essential oils before applying them to a child's skin. A general guideline is to use a 0.5-1% dilution, which equates to 1-2 drops of essential oil per ounce of carrier oil.

3. Carrier Oils: Choose gentle carrier oils like coconut oil, jojoba oil, or sweet almond oil for dilution. Avoid nut-based oils if the child has nut allergies.

4. Patch Test: Perform a patch test on a small area of the child's skin to check for any adverse reactions or sensitivities to the oil blend.

5. Proper Storage: Store essential oils out of children's reach, in a cool, dark place, and with childproof caps. Educate older children about the importance of keeping oils safely stored.

6. Inhalation: Use caution when diffusing essential oils in a child's room. Ensure proper ventilation and use child-friendly diffusers. Limit diffusion time to 30 minutes or less.

Essential Oils Suitable for Children:

1. Lavender (Lavandula angustifolia): Lavender is generally safe for children and can help with sleep, calming, and soothing skin irritations.

2. Chamomile (Chamaemelum nobile or Matricaria chamomilla): Chamomile oil is gentle and can be used to ease anxiety and promote relaxation.

3. Tea Tree (Melaleuca alternifolia): Tea tree oil can be applied topically to address minor skin issues but should be highly diluted.

4. Eucalyptus (Eucalyptus radiata): Eucalyptus can be used with caution for respiratory support in children over two years old. It should be heavily diluted and used sparingly.

Avoid the Following Essential Oils with Children:

1. Peppermint (Mentha piperita): Peppermint oil can be too strong for young children and may cause respiratory distress.

2. Clove (Syzygium aromaticum): Clove oil can irritate the skin and mucous membranes, so it's best avoided.

3. Wintergreen (Gaultheria procumbens): Wintergreen contains methyl salicylate, which can be toxic when ingested. It should not be used with children.

Educate and Supervise:

Teach children about essential oil safety and ensure they understand that essential oils are not to be ingested. Always supervise their use of essential oils, even if they are old enough to apply them independently.

Conclusion: Prioritizing Child Safety with Essential Oils

Using essential oils with children can offer many benefits when done safely and responsibly. By following these essential safety precautions and guidelines, you can create a positive and beneficial experience for your child while minimizing the risk of adverse reactions. Always consult with a qualified aromatherapist or healthcare professional when in doubt, and prioritize the well-being of your child by making informed choices when using essential oils in their daily routine.

The Art of Steam Distillation: Extracting Essential Oils

Introduction:

Essential oils, prized for their aromatic and therapeutic properties, are extracted from various parts of plants, including flowers, leaves, bark, and roots. One of the most common and traditional methods for extracting essential oils is steam distillation. This age-old process involves the careful application of steam to release and capture the precious oils contained within plant material. In this comprehensive text, we will delve into the fascinating world of steam distillation, exploring the art and science behind this time-honored technique.

Steam Distillation: The Essence of Essential Oils

Steam distillation is a process that dates back centuries, with roots in ancient civilizations like Egypt and India. It remains a widely used method due to its effectiveness in extracting essential oils without compromising their purity and potency. Here's an overview of how steam distillation works:

1. Plant Material Selection: The choice of plant material is crucial. Different parts of plants, such as leaves, flowers, or seeds, yield distinct essential oils with unique aromas and therapeutic properties.

2. Steam Generation: Water is heated to produce steam, which serves as a gentle and non-destructive means of extracting essential oils.

3. Steam Passage Through Plant Material: The steam is passed through a chamber containing the plant material. As the steam circulates, it breaks down the oil glands and releases the essential oils.

4. Vapor Condensation: The mixture of steam and essential oil vapor is then passed into a cooling system, where it condenses back into liquid form. The resulting liquid is a combination of water and essential oil.

5. Separation: The water and essential oil are separated, typically through the use of a separator or separator funnel. Essential oils, being less dense than water, float on the surface and are collected.

6. Bottling: The collected essential oil is carefully bottled, sealed, and labeled for distribution and use.

Factors Influencing the Steam Distillation Process:

Several factors can influence the quality and yield of essential oils extracted through steam distillation:

1. Plant Species: Different plant species contain varying amounts and types of essential oils, affecting the final product's aroma and properties.

2. Plant Maturity: The age and maturity of the plant at harvest can impact the oil's composition and aroma.

3. Steam Temperature and Pressure: Adjusting the temperature and pressure of the steam can optimize the extraction process for specific plant materials.

4. Extraction Time: The duration of steam exposure to plant material can vary depending on the plant and the desired oil.

Benefits of Steam Distillation:

1. Purity: Steam distillation is known for producing high-quality, pure essential oils, as it doesn't involve chemical solvents or additives.

2. Therapeutic Properties: Essential oils extracted via steam distillation retain their therapeutic properties, making them suitable for aromatherapy and wellness applications.

3. Aromatic Complexity: This method preserves the complex aroma profiles of essential oils, capturing their full spectrum of fragrances.

Common Essential Oils Extracted by Steam Distillation:

1. Lavender (Lavandula angustifolia): Known for its calming and soothing properties, lavender oil is a staple in aromatherapy.

2. Eucalyptus (Eucalyptus globulus): Eucalyptus oil is renowned for its respiratory benefits and invigorating scent.

3. Peppermint (Mentha piperita): Peppermint oil is valued for its refreshing aroma and digestive support.

4. Tea Tree (Melaleuca alternifolia): Tea tree oil is prized for its antimicrobial properties and skin care benefits.

5. Rosemary (Rosmarinus officinalis): Rosemary oil is known for its cognitive-enhancing properties and herbaceous aroma.

Conclusion: Preserving Nature's Essence with Steam Distillation

Steam distillation is a time-honored technique that allows us to harness the essence of nature, encapsulating the aromatic and therapeutic qualities of plants in the form of essential oils. This process, rooted in tradition and science, continues to be a cornerstone of the essential oil industry. Whether for aromatherapy, natural remedies, or personal care products, essential oils obtained through steam distillation offer a pure and authentic connection to the healing power of plants.

Essential Oils for All-Natural Cleaning: Ditching Harmful Chemicals

Introduction:

The cleaning products we use in our homes can have a significant impact on our health and the environment. Many conventional cleaners contain harsh chemicals that not only pose health risks but also contribute to pollution and harm aquatic life. Fortunately, there's a safer and more eco-friendly way to keep your home clean and fresh – using essential oils. In this text, we'll explore how essential oils can be harnessed for all-natural cleaning, allowing you to ditch harmful chemicals and create a healthier, greener living environment.

The Downsides of Conventional Cleaning Products:

1. Health Risks: Many commercial cleaners contain chemicals like ammonia, bleach, and phthalates, which can irritate the respiratory system and have adverse health effects with prolonged exposure.

2. Environmental Impact: Chemical-laden cleaning products can harm aquatic life and contribute to water pollution when washed down the drain.

3. Asthma Triggers: The fumes from conventional cleaners can exacerbate asthma and allergy symptoms, particularly in children.

The Power of Essential Oils in Cleaning:

Essential oils are derived from plant materials and offer a natural, non-toxic, and effective way to clean and disinfect your home. Here's how essential oils can transform your cleaning routine:

1. Antibacterial and Antiviral Properties: Essential oils like tea tree, lavender, and eucalyptus possess antibacterial and antiviral properties, making them effective at killing germs and preventing the spread of illnesses.

2. Pleasant Aroma: Essential oils infuse your home with delightful natural scents, replacing the artificial fragrances found in commercial cleaners.

3. Non-Toxic: Unlike harsh chemicals, essential oils are safe for you, your family, and the environment.

Essential Oils for All-Natural Cleaning:

1. Lemon (Citrus limon): Lemon oil is an excellent degreaser and can remove stains and odors. It leaves a fresh, citrusy scent.

2. Tea Tree (Melaleuca alternifolia): Tea tree oil is a potent antimicrobial agent and can help disinfect surfaces and eliminate mold and mildew.

3. Lavender (Lavandula angustifolia): Lavender oil is known for its soothing scent and antibacterial properties, making it ideal for gentle cleaning.

4. Peppermint (Mentha piperita): Peppermint oil leaves a refreshing scent and has natural insect-repellent properties.

5. Eucalyptus (Eucalyptus globulus): Eucalyptus oil is effective against bacteria and can help clear the airways, making it suitable for cleaning and supporting respiratory health.

DIY Essential Oil Cleaning Recipes:

1. All-Purpose Cleaner: Mix 1 cup of water, 1 cup of white vinegar, and 15-20 drops of your preferred essential oil (e.g., lavender, lemon, or tea tree) in a spray bottle.

2. Disinfectant Spray: Combine 1 cup of water, 1/2 cup of white vinegar, 10 drops of tea tree oil, and 10 drops of lemon oil in a spray bottle.

3. Natural Air Freshener: Mix 1 cup of water and 10-15 drops of your favorite essential oil (e.g., lavender, peppermint, or eucalyptus) in a spray bottle for a fresh home scent.

Safety Considerations:

- Always store essential oils and cleaning products out of reach of children and pets.

- Test surfaces in an inconspicuous area before using essential oils to ensure they won't cause damage or staining.

Conclusion: A Cleaner, Safer Home with Essential Oils

By harnessing the power of essential oils, you can transform your cleaning routine into a safer and more eco-friendly practice. Say goodbye to harsh chemicals and hello to a healthier home environment. Essential oils not only clean effectively but also leave behind a refreshing, natural fragrance that will make your home a more pleasant place to live. As you embrace the use of essential oils in cleaning, you'll be contributing to a greener and more sustainable future for our planet while prioritizing the well-being of your family and loved ones.

The Connection Between Essential Oils and Dreams

Introduction:

Dreams have fascinated and mystified humans for centuries. They offer a gateway to our subconscious mind, where our deepest thoughts, desires, and fears often manifest. What if there was a way to enhance and explore the world of dreams naturally? Essential oils, with their aromatic and therapeutic qualities, have been used for centuries to support various aspects of well-being, including sleep and dream experiences. In this comprehensive text, we'll delve into the intriguing connection between essential oils and dreams, exploring how these aromatic compounds can influence our nighttime journeys into the subconscious.

Understanding Dreams:

Before we dive into the role of essential oils in dream enhancement, let's briefly explore the fascinating realm of dreams:

1. Subconscious Exploration: Dreams offer a unique opportunity to explore the subconscious mind, where thoughts, emotions, and memories often surface in symbolic or abstract forms.

2. Dream Types: Dreams come in various forms, including lucid dreams (where the dreamer is aware they are dreaming), vivid dreams,

recurring dreams, and prophetic dreams (which seem to predict future events).

3. Emotional Processing: Dreams can serve as a tool for emotional processing, helping us work through unresolved issues, fears, and anxieties.

The Power of Aromatherapy:

Aromatherapy, the use of essential oils for therapeutic purposes, has gained recognition for its potential to influence mood, emotions, and even sleep quality. The connection between essential oils and dreams lies in the way certain scents can create an environment conducive to relaxation and a heightened dream state.

Essential Oils for Dream Enhancement:

1. Lavender (Lavandula angustifolia): Lavender oil is renowned for its calming properties. Inhaling lavender before sleep can induce a peaceful state of mind, potentially leading to more tranquil dreams.

2. Chamomile (Chamaemelum nobile or Matricaria chamomilla): Chamomile oil's soothing aroma can help reduce anxiety and promote relaxation, fostering an environment for pleasant dreams.

3. Sandalwood (Santalum album): Sandalwood oil has a grounding and spiritually enhancing scent, which can contribute to more profound dream experiences.

4. Cedarwood (Cedrus atlantica): Cedarwood's earthy fragrance can evoke a sense of security and stability, potentially influencing the content of dreams.

5. Clary Sage (Salvia sclarea): Clary sage oil is known for its ability to stimulate vivid and lucid dreaming experiences.

Practical Application:

1. Diffusion: Diffuse essential oils in your bedroom before sleep using an essential oil diffuser. This creates an aromatic environment that encourages relaxation and dream enhancement.

2. Topical Application: Dilute essential oils in a carrier oil and apply a small amount to your pulse points, such as wrists and neck, before bedtime.

3. Aromatic Baths: Add a few drops of essential oil to a warm bath before sleep to envelop yourself in the soothing scent.

4. Dream Journal: Keep a dream journal by your bedside to record your dreams upon waking. Over time, you may notice patterns or connections between certain oils and dream experiences.

Safety Considerations:

- Always use high-quality, pure essential oils to ensure safety and efficacy.
- Use essential oils in moderation and according to recommended dilution guidelines.
- Be aware of any personal sensitivities or allergies to specific oils.

Conclusion: Enhancing Dreamscapes with Essential Oils

The world of dreams is a captivating and mysterious realm that has intrigued humans for generations. Essential oils, with their ability to influence mood and relaxation, can serve as a natural and gentle tool for enhancing dream experiences. By incorporating the power of aromatherapy into your bedtime routine, you may find that your dreams become more vivid, meaningful, and enjoyable. As you explore the connection between essential oils and dreams, you embark on a journey into the depths of your subconscious, uncovering hidden insights and emotions along the way. Sweet dreams await, filled with the enchanting scents of essential oils.

Tea Tree Oil: A Natural Antiseptic and Skin Healer

Introduction:

Tea tree oil, derived from the leaves of the Australian tea tree (Melaleuca alternifolia), has earned a well-deserved reputation as a versatile and potent essential oil. For centuries, it has been used by indigenous Australian communities for its remarkable healing properties. Today, tea tree oil is celebrated worldwide for its natural antiseptic, antibacterial, and skin-healing abilities. In this comprehensive text, we'll explore the fascinating history, science, and practical applications of tea tree oil in promoting skin health and overall well-being.

A Brief History of Tea Tree Oil:

The use of tea tree oil can be traced back thousands of years to the indigenous people of Australia. They discovered that the leaves of the tea tree had powerful medicinal properties, using them to treat various ailments and infections. The knowledge of tea tree oil eventually made its way to European settlers, who recognized its therapeutic potential.

Tea Tree Oil's Key Components:

Tea tree oil owes its remarkable healing properties to a unique combination of bioactive compounds, including:

1. Terpinen-4-ol: This is the primary antimicrobial component responsible for tea tree oil's antiseptic and antibacterial properties.

2. 1,8-Cineole: Known for its anti-inflammatory and analgesic effects, it helps reduce pain and inflammation.

3. Alpha-Pinene: An anti-inflammatory compound that also contributes to the oil's fresh, pine-like scent.

Natural Antiseptic and Antibacterial Properties:

One of tea tree oil's most celebrated qualities is its natural antiseptic and antibacterial action. It can:

- Combat Skin Infections: Tea tree oil effectively kills bacteria, fungi, and viruses, making it valuable for treating various skin infections, including acne, athlete's foot, and nail fungus.

- Reduce Acne: Its antimicrobial properties help unclog pores and reduce acne breakouts. It also reduces inflammation and redness associated with acne.

- Relieve Skin Irritations: Tea tree oil can soothe itching, redness, and irritation caused by insect bites, rashes, and minor burns.

Skin Healing and Regeneration:

In addition to its antimicrobial properties, tea tree oil supports the skin's natural healing processes. It can:

- Promote Wound Healing: Tea tree oil accelerates the healing of minor cuts, abrasions, and wounds by stimulating the production of collagen, the protein responsible for skin repair.

- Reduce Scarring: By aiding in proper wound healing, tea tree oil may reduce the appearance of scars.

- Moisturize Dry Skin: It helps alleviate dryness and flakiness by locking in moisture and restoring the skin's natural balance.

Practical Applications:

1. Acne Spot Treatment: Dab a drop of tea tree oil onto a cotton swab and apply it directly to acne spots.

2. Antifungal Foot Soak: Add a few drops of tea tree oil to warm water for a soothing foot soak to combat athlete's foot or nail fungus.

3. Skin Toner: Mix a few drops of tea tree oil with water or aloe vera gel and apply it as a toner to balance oily skin and prevent acne.

4. First Aid Kit Essential: Include tea tree oil in your first aid kit for on-the-go relief from minor skin irritations and insect bites.

Safety Considerations:

- Always dilute tea tree oil with carrier oil (e.g., coconut oil, jojoba oil) before applying it to the skin, as it can be irritating when used undiluted.

- Perform a patch test before applying tea tree oil to a larger area to check for any adverse reactions or sensitivities.

Conclusion: Nature's Skin Healer in a Bottle

Tea tree oil's natural antiseptic and skin-healing properties have made it a beloved and invaluable addition to skincare routines worldwide. From combating acne to soothing insect bites, this versatile essential oil offers a gentle and effective solution for various skin concerns. As you incorporate tea tree oil into your daily regimen, you harness the healing power of nature to promote clear, healthy, and radiant skin. Embrace the centuries-old wisdom of indigenous cultures and let tea tree oil become your go-to remedy for skin health and overall well-being.

Essential Oils for Emotional Release: Letting Go of Negativity

Introduction:

Emotions are an integral part of the human experience, influencing our thoughts, behaviors, and overall well-being. Sometimes, we may find ourselves holding onto negative emotions like stress, anger, or sadness, which can impact our mental and emotional health. Essential oils, with their aromatic and therapeutic properties, can play a powerful role in helping us release and manage these emotions. In this comprehensive text, we'll explore the world of essential oils for emotional release, offering insights into how these natural remedies can support us on our journey toward greater emotional well-being.

Understanding Emotional Release:

Emotional release is the process of acknowledging, processing, and letting go of pent-up or negative emotions. This can be essential for maintaining mental and emotional balance. When we suppress or ignore emotions, they can manifest in various ways, affecting our mental health, relationships, and overall quality of life.

The Role of Essential Oils:

Essential oils have been used for centuries in aromatherapy for their potential to influence mood and emotions. Here's how they can assist in emotional release:

1. Aromatic Influence: Inhaling the aroma of essential oils can stimulate the limbic system, the brain's emotional center, triggering emotional responses and memories.

2. Emotional Balancing: Many essential oils possess properties that can help balance and stabilize emotions, reducing the impact of negative feelings.

3. Relaxation: Certain essential oils have a calming effect on the nervous system, promoting relaxation and reducing stress.

Essential Oils for Emotional Release:

1. Lavender (Lavandula angustifolia): Lavender oil is renowned for its calming properties, making it an excellent choice for reducing stress and anxiety.

2. Frankincense (Boswellia carterii): Frankincense oil promotes feelings of peace and relaxation, making it useful for emotional grounding.

3. Chamomile (Chamaemelum nobile): Chamomile oil soothes and calms the mind, helping release tension and negativity.

4. Ylang-Ylang (Cananga odorata): Ylang-ylang oil is known for its uplifting and euphoric qualities, making it effective for combating sadness and promoting joy.

5. Bergamot (Citrus bergamia): Bergamot oil has a bright and uplifting scent, which can help alleviate stress and promote positivity.

Practical Application:

1. Diffusion: Use an essential oil diffuser to disperse the aroma of your chosen oil throughout your space.

2. Aromatherapy Jewelry: Wear aromatherapy jewelry, such as diffuser necklaces or bracelets, to carry the scent of essential oils with you throughout the day.

3. Topical Application: Dilute essential oils in a carrier oil and apply them to pulse points like wrists or temples for a calming effect.

4. Bathing: Add a few drops of essential oil to a warm bath for a soothing and therapeutic soak.

Emotional Release Ritual:

Create a calming and intentional ritual using essential oils:

1. Find a quiet and comfortable space where you won't be disturbed.

2. Choose an essential oil that resonates with your emotional needs in the moment.

3. Inhale deeply while holding the bottle of essential oil to your nose.

4. Close your eyes, take slow, deep breaths, and focus on the aroma, allowing it to evoke positive emotions and release negativity.

5. Visualize letting go of any emotional baggage, imagining it dissipating like a cloud.

6. After a few moments, open your eyes, feeling refreshed and emotionally lighter.

Conclusion: Embracing Emotional Freedom with Essential Oils

The journey toward emotional release and well-being is a personal and transformative one. Essential oils, with their natural and aromatic properties, can be invaluable companions on this path. By incorporating them into your daily routine and practicing intentional rituals, you can create a space for emotional healing and growth. As you let go of negativity and embrace positive emotions, you empower yourself to live a more balanced and joyful life. Essential oils become not just fragrant elixirs but powerful tools for emotional release and greater well-being.

Sandalwood Essential Oil: A Sacred Scent in Spiritual Practices

Introduction:

Sandalwood, revered for centuries for its rich and sacred aroma, holds a special place in the world of spirituality and holistic well-being. Derived from the heartwood of the sandalwood tree (Santalum album), sandalwood essential oil is known for its deeply grounding, meditative, and spiritually uplifting properties. In this comprehensive text, we'll explore the profound connection between sandalwood essential oil and spiritual practices, shedding light on its history, significance, and practical applications in fostering a deeper sense of inner peace and spiritual connection.

The History of Sandalwood:

The use of sandalwood dates back thousands of years, with its origins deeply rooted in ancient India. It has played a significant role in Hindu, Buddhist, and other spiritual and religious traditions. Sandalwood was considered a sacred offering to deities, a symbol of purification, and an aid in meditation.

Spiritual Significance:

Sandalwood essential oil is esteemed for its spiritual and metaphysical properties:

1. Grounding: Sandalwood's earthy and woody scent promotes a sense of grounding, helping individuals feel centered and connected to the present moment.

2. Meditation: Its aroma is conducive to deep meditation, facilitating inner reflection and spiritual exploration.

3. Spiritual Cleansing: Sandalwood is believed to clear negative energy and create a sacred space for spiritual practices.

4. Balancing: It can help balance emotions, providing emotional stability during times of stress or inner turmoil.

Practical Applications:

1. Meditation: Diffuse sandalwood essential oil during meditation to create a serene and sacred atmosphere. Apply a drop to your third eye (forehead) or heart chakra for enhanced spiritual experiences.

2. Spiritual Rituals: Use sandalwood oil as a component of spiritual rituals, such as prayer, mantra recitation, or offering to deities.

3. Aromatherapy Jewelry: Wear a sandalwood bead bracelet or necklace infused with sandalwood essential oil to carry the aroma with you throughout the day.

4. Bathing: Add a few drops of sandalwood oil to your bath for a deeply relaxing and spiritually rejuvenating soak.

Chakras and Sandalwood:

Sandalwood essential oil is associated with the crown chakra (Sahasrara) and the root chakra (Muladhara). Here's how it interacts with these energy centers:

1. Crown Chakra: Sandalwood's grounding properties can help align the crown chakra, promoting a sense of spiritual connectedness and enlightenment.

2. Root Chakra: Sandalwood's earthy scent can anchor the root chakra, providing a sense of security and stability during spiritual practices.

Safety Considerations:

- Sandalwood essential oil is generally safe for topical use when properly diluted. However, it is a precious and potent oil, so a little goes a long way.

- Ensure that you purchase high-quality, pure sandalwood oil from a reputable source.

Conclusion: Elevating the Spirit with Sandalwood

Sandalwood essential oil, with its deep-rooted history and spiritual significance, has been a cherished companion on the spiritual journey for countless individuals. Its grounding, meditative, and emotionally balancing properties make it a valuable tool for anyone seeking a deeper connection with themselves and the spiritual realm. Whether used in meditation, rituals, or as part of daily aromatherapy, sandalwood oil has the power to elevate the spirit and create a sacred space for inner exploration and spiritual growth. As you embrace the sacred scent of sandalwood, you embark on a journey of self-discovery, inner peace, and spiritual enlightenment guided by the profound wisdom of this revered essential oil.

The Benefits of Essential Oils for Oral Health

Introduction:

Oral health is an essential aspect of overall well-being, with a direct impact on our daily lives. While regular dental care practices like brushing, flossing, and dental check-ups are crucial, there's another natural and holistic approach that can enhance your oral health journey: essential oils. Derived from aromatic plant materials, essential oils offer a wide range of benefits for oral hygiene, from combating bad breath to promoting healthy gums and teeth. In this comprehensive text, we'll explore the numerous advantages of using essential oils for oral health, shedding light on their history, effectiveness, and practical applications in maintaining a radiant smile.

The Historical Use of Essential Oils for Oral Care:

The use of essential oils in oral hygiene can be traced back thousands of years to various cultures around the world. Ancient civilizations, such as the Egyptians, Greeks, and Romans, utilized essential oils for their natural antiseptic, antibacterial, and aromatic properties. These oils were employed in mouthwashes, toothpaste-like preparations, and as breath fresheners.

The Benefits of Essential Oils for Oral Health:

1. Antibacterial Properties: Many essential oils, such as tea tree, peppermint, and clove, possess potent antibacterial properties that can combat the bacteria responsible for gum disease, cavities, and bad breath.

2. Anti-Inflammatory Effects: Certain essential oils, like lavender and chamomile, have anti-inflammatory properties that can help reduce gum inflammation and soothe oral discomfort.

3. Fresh Breath: Essential oils like peppermint, spearmint, and cinnamon are known for their refreshing and long-lasting breath-freshening qualities.

4. Promoting Healthy Gums: Regular use of essential oils can support gum health by reducing inflammation, fighting bacteria, and promoting proper circulation.

Practical Applications:

1. Natural Mouthwash: Create a natural mouthwash by diluting a few drops of essential oil (e.g., tea tree, peppermint) in water. Swish it around your mouth for 30 seconds, then spit it out.

2. DIY Toothpaste: Make your own toothpaste by mixing baking soda, coconut oil, and a few drops of an essential oil (e.g., peppermint, clove) to clean and freshen your teeth.

3. Gum Massage: Dilute an essential oil (e.g., lavender, chamomile) in a carrier oil and gently massage it into your gums for soothing relief.

4. Breath Freshener: Carry a small bottle of breath-freshening essential oil (e.g., peppermint, spearmint) and inhale it when needed for instant freshness.

Safety Considerations:

- Always use high-quality, pure essential oils from reputable sources.

- Essential oils are potent, so they should be diluted with a carrier oil before applying directly to the skin or mouth.

- Some essential oils can be toxic if ingested in large amounts, so avoid swallowing mouthwash or toothpaste containing essential oils.

Conclusion: Nurturing Your Oral Health Naturally

Essential oils offer a natural and holistic approach to oral health that can complement traditional dental care practices. Their antibacterial, anti-inflammatory, and breath-freshening properties make them valuable allies in maintaining a healthy smile. As you incorporate essential oils into your daily oral care routine, you not only support your dental health but also enjoy the aromatic pleasures of nature's remedies. With the wisdom of ancient civilizations and the effectiveness of modern science, essential oils become a holistic and refreshing way to nurture your oral well-being, one drop at a time.

Citrus Oils: Energizing, Uplifting, and Refreshing Scents

Introduction:

Citrus oils are among the most beloved and widely used essential oils in aromatherapy and natural wellness practices. Derived from the peels of citrus fruits like oranges, lemons, limes, and grapefruits, these oils are celebrated for their bright and invigorating aromas. Citrus oils are well-known for their ability to uplift the spirits, boost energy levels, and promote a sense of vitality and well-being. In this comprehensive text, we'll delve into the world of citrus essential oils, exploring their origins, therapeutic benefits, and practical applications for enhancing your daily life.

The Rich History of Citrus Oils:

Citrus fruits, native to Southeast Asia, have been cultivated for centuries and have played a significant role in culinary, medicinal, and aromatic traditions. Essential oils extracted from citrus peels have been used in traditional medicine, perfumery, and as natural flavorings for food and beverages.

The Therapeutic Benefits of Citrus Oils:

Citrus essential oils are celebrated for their wide-ranging therapeutic benefits:

1. Mood Elevation: Citrus oils, such as sweet orange and bergamot, have natural mood-enhancing properties that can help reduce stress, anxiety, and symptoms of depression.

2. Energy Boost: The invigorating scents of citrus oils are known to increase alertness, mental clarity, and energy levels. They make excellent choices for combating fatigue and boosting motivation.

3. Immune Support: Citrus oils are rich in antioxidants and vitamin C, which can support the immune system and help ward off colds and infections.

4. Refreshing Aromas: The fresh, zesty scents of citrus oils can instantly refresh and revitalize any space, making them ideal for creating a lively and inviting atmosphere.

Popular Citrus Essential Oils:

1. Sweet Orange (Citrus sinensis): Known for its sweet and cheerful aroma, sweet orange oil is an excellent mood-lifter and energizer.

2. Lemon (Citrus limon): Lemon oil has a bright and zesty scent that promotes mental clarity and focus. It's also a powerful natural cleaner.

3. Lime (Citrus aurantiifolia): Lime oil's crisp aroma is both uplifting and refreshing, making it a go-to choice for revitalizing blends.

4. Grapefruit (Citrus paradisi): Grapefruit oil has a lively and citrusy scent that can help reduce cravings and promote weight management.

5. Bergamot (Citrus bergamia): Bergamot oil has a unique, floral-citrus scent that soothes the nerves and supports emotional balance.

Practical Applications:

1. Diffusion: Add a few drops of citrus oil to an essential oil diffuser to fill your space with a refreshing and invigorating aroma.

2. Inhalation: Inhale directly from the bottle or add a drop to a tissue for a quick mood boost.

3. Massage: Dilute citrus oils in a carrier oil and use them for a rejuvenating and uplifting massage.

4. DIY Cleaning: Mix citrus oils with vinegar and water to create a natural and effective cleaning solution for your home.

Safety Considerations:

- Citrus oils are phototoxic, so avoid applying them to your skin if you'll be exposed to direct sunlight.

- Store citrus oils in a cool, dark place to preserve their freshness and potency.

Conclusion: Embrace the Zest for Life with Citrus Oils

Citrus essential oils offer a vibrant and aromatic approach to enhancing your mood, boosting your energy, and infusing your surroundings with a sense of freshness and vitality. From the sunny groves of citrus trees to the modern homes and wellness practices of today, these oils continue to brighten and uplift our lives. As you incorporate citrus oils into your daily routines and rituals, you invite the essence of citrus fruits into your life, embracing the zest for life, one drop at a time.

Essential Oils for Pain Relief: Managing Discomfort Naturally

Introduction:

Pain is a universal experience, ranging from everyday aches and discomfort to more persistent and chronic conditions. While modern medicine offers various treatments, essential oils provide a natural and holistic approach to managing pain and promoting well-being. Derived from aromatic plants, these oils offer a wide array of therapeutic benefits, including pain relief. In this comprehensive text, we will explore the world of essential oils for pain relief, delving into their history, efficacy, and practical applications for managing discomfort naturally.

A Brief History of Essential Oils for Pain Relief:

The use of essential oils for pain relief can be traced back to ancient civilizations, where aromatic plants were employed for their analgesic and anti-inflammatory properties. These natural remedies were utilized to alleviate various forms of pain, from headaches and muscle soreness to joint discomfort.

The Mechanism of Pain Relief with Essential Oils:

Essential oils offer pain relief through several mechanisms:

1. Anti-Inflammatory Properties: Many essential oils possess anti-inflammatory properties, helping to reduce inflammation, a common source of pain.

2. Analgesic Effects: Certain essential oils have analgesic properties, which can alleviate pain by dulling pain signals to the brain.

3. Relaxation and Stress Reduction: Essential oils can promote relaxation and reduce stress, which can indirectly alleviate pain caused or exacerbated by tension.

4. Improved Circulation: Some essential oils stimulate circulation, which can enhance the body's natural healing processes.

Essential Oils for Pain Relief:

1. Lavender (Lavandula angustifolia): Lavender oil is known for its calming properties and can help alleviate tension headaches and muscle soreness.

2. Peppermint (Mentha × piperita): Peppermint oil has a cooling sensation and is effective for relieving headaches, migraines, and muscle pain.

3. Eucalyptus (Eucalyptus globulus): Eucalyptus oil's anti-inflammatory properties make it ideal for soothing respiratory discomfort and muscle pain.

4. Chamomile (Chamaemelum nobile): Chamomile oil is well-suited for reducing inflammation and calming nerve-related pain.

5. Frankincense (Boswellia carterii): Frankincense oil promotes relaxation and can ease joint pain and inflammation.

Practical Applications:

1. Topical Application: Dilute essential oils in a carrier oil (e.g., coconut, jojoba) and apply the mixture to the affected area for localized pain relief.

2. Aromatherapy: Inhale the aroma of essential oils using a diffuser or by adding a few drops to a bowl of hot water.

3. Massage: Incorporate essential oils into a massage oil blend for a relaxing and pain-relieving massage.

4. Compress: Create a warm or cold compress by adding essential oils to a bowl of water, soaking a cloth, and applying it to the painful area.

5. Bathing: Add a few drops of essential oils to a warm bath to soothe sore muscles and promote relaxation.

Safety Considerations:

- Always dilute essential oils before applying them to the skin, as they can be irritating when used undiluted.

- Perform a patch test before applying essential oils to a larger area to check for any adverse reactions or sensitivities.

- Consult with a healthcare professional, especially if you have a chronic or serious medical condition, before using essential oils for pain relief.

Conclusion: Embracing Natural Pain Relief with Essential Oils

Essential oils offer a natural and holistic approach to pain relief, allowing you to manage discomfort while nurturing your well-being. Whether you're dealing with headaches, muscle soreness, joint pain, or other forms of discomfort, essential oils can be valuable allies on your journey to feeling your best. As you incorporate these aromatic remedies into your daily life, you embrace the power of nature to soothe and heal, naturally and holistically. Essential oils become not just fragrant elixirs but effective tools for managing pain and promoting a higher quality of life, one drop at a time.

Palo Santo Essential Oil: Purifying and Cleansing Properties

Introduction:

Palo Santo, a sacred wood native to South America, has been revered for centuries for its spiritual and purifying qualities. The essential oil extracted from Palo Santo wood carries these remarkable properties, making it a valuable tool for cleansing and revitalizing the mind, body, and spirit. In this comprehensive text, we'll explore the world of Palo Santo essential oil, uncovering its origins, cultural significance, therapeutic benefits, and practical applications for harnessing its purifying and cleansing power.

The Origins and Cultural Significance of Palo Santo:

Palo Santo, which translates to "holy wood" in Spanish, comes from the wood of the Bursera graveolens tree, primarily found in the coastal regions of South America, particularly Peru and Ecuador. It has a rich history deeply intertwined with indigenous traditions and shamanic rituals.

The Therapeutic Benefits of Palo Santo Essential Oil:

Palo Santo essential oil boasts an array of therapeutic benefits:

1. Spiritual Cleansing: Palo Santo oil is renowned for its ability to purify and cleanse energy, making it a valuable tool for spiritual rituals and meditation.

2. Emotional Balance: Its grounding and calming aroma can help alleviate stress, anxiety, and emotional turmoil, promoting a sense of inner peace.

3. Respiratory Support: Palo Santo oil can support respiratory health by soothing coughs and congestion when diffused or inhaled.

4. Pain Relief: It has mild analgesic properties, which can help ease headaches, muscle pain, and inflammation when applied topically.

Practical Applications:

1. Aromatherapy: Diffuse Palo Santo essential oil in an essential oil diffuser to cleanse and purify the energy in your space. Its woody and resinous aroma promotes relaxation and focus.

2. Topical Application: Dilute Palo Santo oil in a carrier oil (e.g., jojoba or coconut oil) and apply it to the wrists, temples, or the back of the neck for emotional and physical support.

3. Spiritual Rituals: Palo Santo oil is often used in spiritual ceremonies, rituals, and smudging practices to clear negative energy and invite positivity.

4. Meditation: Enhance your meditation sessions by diffusing Palo Santo oil or applying it to pulse points to create a sacred and calming atmosphere.

Safety Considerations:

- Palo Santo essential oil is generally safe when used in moderation and properly diluted. Always dilute it in a carrier oil before applying it to the skin.

- Consult with a healthcare professional if you are pregnant, nursing, have a medical condition or are taking medication before using Palo Santo oil.

Conclusion: Embrace the Cleansing Power of Palo Santo

Palo Santo essential oil, with its rich history and profound spiritual significance, offers a natural and holistic way to cleanse and purify your mind, body, and surroundings. Whether you seek to enhance your spiritual practice, reduce stress, or simply create a sense of peace and well-being, Palo Santo oil can be a valuable addition to your holistic wellness toolkit. As you incorporate this sacred and aromatic remedy into your daily life, you connect with centuries of tradition and wisdom, embracing the cleansing power of Palo Santo to uplift and revitalize your being, one drop at a time.

Creating Custom Essential Oil Perfumes for Mood Enhancement

Introduction:

The art of crafting custom essential oil perfumes is a delightful and personal way to harness the therapeutic properties of aromatherapy. By blending various essential oils, you can create fragrances that not only smell captivating but also have the power to enhance your mood and well-being. In this comprehensive text, we'll explore the fascinating world of creating custom essential oil perfumes, guiding you through the process, discussing the benefits, and offering some mood-enhancing perfume recipes to inspire your olfactory journey.

Why Create Custom Essential Oil Perfumes?

1. Personalized Aromatherapy: Custom perfumes allow you to tailor your scent to your specific emotional and therapeutic needs.

2. Chemical-Free Fragrance: Homemade perfumes contain no synthetic chemicals or harmful additives often found in commercial fragrances.

3. Mood Enhancement: Certain essential oils can have a profound impact on your mood, helping you feel relaxed, uplifted, or focused.

How to Create Custom Essential Oil Perfumes:

Ingredients:

- A selection of high-quality essential oils (base, middle, and top notes)
- A carrier oil (e.g., jojoba, sweet almond oil)
- A glass perfume bottle or rollerball bottle
- A small funnel
- A glass dropper

Steps:

1. Choose Your Base Note: Base notes are the foundation of your perfume and typically include deep, long-lasting scents. Examples include cedarwood, patchouli, and sandalwood.

2. Select Middle Notes: Middle notes provide a harmonious bridge between the base and top notes. Options include lavender, rosemary, and ylang-ylang.

3. Add Top Notes: Top notes are the initial fragrances that greet your senses and tend to be light and refreshing. These can include citrus oils like lemon, bergamot, and sweet orange.

4. Dilute in Carrier Oil: Using a small funnel, combine your chosen essential oils in the glass perfume bottle. Fill the bottle about halfway

with your carrier oil, and then add your essential oil blend. Leave some space at the top for shaking.

5. Shake and Age: Cap the bottle and shake it gently to mix the oils. Let the perfume age for at least a week in a cool, dark place to allow the scents to meld and mature.

6. Test and Adjust: After aging, test your perfume on your wrist and adjust the blend if needed. You can add more essential oils or carrier oil to achieve your desired scent.

7. Label and Store: Label your custom perfume bottle with the date and ingredients. Store it in a cool, dark place to preserve the fragrance.

Mood-Enhancing Perfume Recipes:

1. Calming Lavender Dream:
   - Base Note: Cedarwood
   - Middle Note: Lavender
   - Top Note: Bergamot

2. Uplifting Citrus Bliss:
   - Base Note: Sandalwood
   - Middle Note: Ylang-ylang

- Top Note: Lemon

3. Focus and Clarity:
   - Base Note: Patchouli
   - Middle Note: Rosemary
   - Top Note: Peppermint

Safety Considerations:

- Perform a patch test on your skin to check for allergies or sensitivities to the essential oils used.

- Always dilute essential oils in a carrier oil to prevent skin irritation.

Conclusion: Express Yourself Through Scent

Creating custom essential oil perfumes is a beautiful way to infuse your daily life with the therapeutic benefits of aromatherapy. Each fragrance you craft becomes a personal expression of your emotions, intentions, and well-being. As you embark on this aromatic journey, you not only enjoy delightful scents but also enhance your mood and elevate your spirit through the power of natural essential oils. Embrace the art of custom perfume making, and let your unique blend become a fragrant reflection of your inner self.

The Impact of Essential Oils on Mood Disorders like Depression and Anxiety

Introduction:

Mood disorders, such as depression and anxiety, affect millions of individuals worldwide, often taking a toll on their emotional well-being and quality of life. While conventional treatments exist, many people seek complementary and holistic approaches to manage these conditions. Essential oils, derived from aromatic plants, have gained recognition for their potential to alleviate symptoms of mood disorders and promote emotional balance. In this comprehensive text, we'll delve into the world of essential oils and their impact on mood disorders, exploring their historical use, scientific evidence, and practical applications for those seeking natural relief.

Historical Use of Essential Oils for Mood Disorders:

The use of essential oils to address emotional and mental well-being has deep historical roots. Ancient civilizations, including the Egyptians and Greeks, recognized the therapeutic value of aromatic plant extracts in promoting emotional balance and inner harmony. These oils were used in rituals, massages, and aromatherapy practices to lift spirits and soothe troubled minds.

Scientific Evidence and Essential Oils:

1. Lavender Oil: Lavender essential oil has been extensively studied for its calming and anxiety-reducing effects. Research suggests that inhaling lavender oil can reduce anxiety levels and improve mood.

2. Frankincense Oil: Frankincense essential oil has shown promise in reducing symptoms of anxiety and depression. It may help regulate emotions and reduce stress.

3. Chamomile Oil: Chamomile essential oil, particularly Roman chamomile, is known for its soothing properties. It can help alleviate symptoms of anxiety and improve sleep quality.

4. Ylang-Ylang Oil: Ylang-ylang essential oil is believed to have a positive impact on mood and may help reduce symptoms of depression and anxiety.

Practical Applications:

1. Aromatherapy: Diffuse essential oils using an essential oil diffuser to create a calming and mood-enhancing atmosphere in your home.

2. Topical Application: Dilute essential oils in a carrier oil and apply them to pulse points, such as the wrists and temples, for emotional support throughout the day.

3. Bathing: Add a few drops of essential oil to a warm bath to relax and soothe your mind.

4. Massage: Incorporate essential oils into a massage oil blend to ease tension and promote relaxation.

Safety Considerations:

- Essential oils are potent and should be used with care. Always dilute them in a carrier oil before applying to the skin.

- Perform a patch test before using any essential oil topically to check for allergies or sensitivities.

- Consult with a healthcare professional if you have a diagnosed mood disorder or are taking medications, as essential oils are complementary and not a substitute for medical treatment.

Conclusion: Nurturing Emotional Well-Being Naturally

Essential oils offer a natural and holistic approach to supporting emotional well-being for those dealing with mood disorders like depression and anxiety. While they may not replace conventional treatments, they can complement therapy and provide a sense of balance and tranquility. As you explore the world of aromatherapy and essential oils, you embark on a journey to nurture your emotional health naturally. Embrace the power of nature's aromatic remedies and allow essential oils to become valuable tools in your quest for emotional harmony and well-being.

Coping with Seasonal Depression Using Aromatherapy

Introduction:

Seasonal depression, also known as Seasonal Affective Disorder (SAD), is a type of depression that occurs seasonally, typically during the fall and winter months when daylight hours are shorter. It can bring about feelings of sadness, fatigue, and a lack of energy, impacting one's overall well-being. While there are various treatments available, including therapy and medication, aromatherapy can be a valuable complementary approach to coping with seasonal depression. In this detailed text, we will explore the concept of seasonal depression, the role of aromatherapy, and practical ways to use essential oils to uplift your mood during the dark and gloomy seasons.

Understanding Seasonal Depression:

Seasonal depression is characterized by the following symptoms:

- Persistent feelings of sadness or hopelessness
- Loss of interest in activities you once enjoyed
- Changes in sleep patterns (oversleeping or insomnia)
- Weight gain or loss
- Fatigue and low energy

- Difficulty concentrating and making decisions

The Role of Aromatherapy in Coping:

Aromatherapy, a holistic approach to well-being, harnesses the therapeutic properties of essential oils to promote mental and emotional balance. Essential oils are derived from aromatic plants and can have a profound impact on mood and overall mental health. When used mindfully, they can help alleviate symptoms of seasonal depression and provide a sense of comfort and relief.

Essential Oils for Seasonal Depression:

1. Lavender (Lavandula angustifolia): Lavender oil is renowned for its calming properties, making it effective in reducing anxiety and promoting relaxation.

2. Bergamot (Citrus bergamia): Bergamot oil has a bright, citrusy aroma that can help elevate mood and reduce feelings of sadness.

3. Frankincense (Boswellia carterii): Frankincense oil is grounding and can promote feelings of inner peace and emotional balance.

4. Geranium (Pelargonium graveolens): Geranium oil is known for its uplifting qualities and can help combat feelings of fatigue and low energy.

5. Orange (Citrus sinensis): Orange oil has a cheerful and invigorating scent, which can boost mood and motivation.

Practical Aromatherapy Techniques:

1. Diffusion: Use an essential oil diffuser to disperse mood-enhancing essential oils into your living space. This can create a calming and uplifting atmosphere.

2. Topical Application: Dilute essential oils in a carrier oil and apply them to pulse points, such as the wrists and temples, for on-the-go emotional support.

3. Bathing: Add a few drops of essential oil to a warm bath to relax and soothe your mind. This can be particularly helpful on dark, cold days.

4. Inhalation: Inhale the aroma of essential oils directly from the bottle or by adding a drop to a tissue. This can provide an immediate mood boost.

Creating a Seasonal Depression Aromatherapy Routine:

- Set aside time each day for aromatherapy, such as a morning diffusing session or a bedtime relaxation ritual.

- Experiment with different essential oils and blends to discover what works best for your mood and preferences.

- Practice mindfulness while inhaling the scents of essential oils, focusing on your breath and the sensations in your body.

Conclusion: Brightening Your Season with Aromatherapy

Coping with seasonal depression can be challenging, but incorporating aromatherapy into your daily routine can provide a natural and uplifting way to support your mental and emotional well-being. As you explore the world of essential oils and their mood-enhancing properties, you can take steps to brighten your season and embrace the comfort and relief that aromatherapy offers. Remember that aromatherapy is a complementary approach, and if you're experiencing severe symptoms of depression, it's essential to seek professional help. With mindfulness and the power of nature's scents, you can find moments of warmth and joy even during the darkest seasons.

Essential Oils for Focus and Concentration During Study and Work

Introduction:

Maintaining focus and concentration during study and work is a common challenge faced by many. Distractions, fatigue, and mental fog can hinder productivity and hinder one's ability to perform at their best. Fortunately, aromatherapy offers a natural and effective solution to enhance focus and concentration. In this detailed text, we will explore the world of essential oils and their role in promoting mental clarity, improving concentration, and boosting productivity during study and work sessions.

Understanding the Challenges of Focus and Concentration:

Achieving and sustaining focus and concentration can be difficult due to several factors:

- Distractions from electronic devices, noise, or interruptions
- Mental fatigue and lack of energy
- Stress and anxiety affecting cognitive function
- Monotony and boredom leading to decreased attention span

The Role of Essential Oils in Enhancing Focus:

Aromatherapy, the practice of using essential oils, can help improve focus and concentration through several mechanisms:

- Aromas and Brain Function: Certain scents have been shown to stimulate the brain and improve cognitive performance.

- Stress Reduction: Essential oils can reduce stress and anxiety, which can cloud thinking and hinder concentration.

- Emotional Balance: Aromatherapy can promote emotional well-being, helping to create a positive and focused mindset.

Essential Oils for Focus and Concentration:

1. Peppermint (Mentha × piperita): Peppermint oil has invigorating properties that can increase alertness and mental clarity.

2. Rosemary (Rosmarinus officinalis): Rosemary oil is known for its cognitive-enhancing effects and can help improve memory and concentration.

3. Lemon (Citrus limon): Lemon oil has a refreshing and uplifting scent that can boost mood and mental focus.

4. Eucalyptus (Eucalyptus globulus): Eucalyptus oil can clear the mind and enhance alertness and productivity.

5. Lavender (Lavandula angustifolia): Lavender oil promotes relaxation and can help reduce stress and mental clutter, improving concentration.

Practical Applications:

1. Diffusion: Use an essential oil diffuser to disperse focus-enhancing essential oils into your workspace. This creates a conducive environment for productivity.

2. Topical Application: Dilute essential oils in a carrier oil and apply them to pulse points, such as the wrists and temples, for on-the-go concentration support.

3. Inhalation: Inhale the aroma of essential oils directly from the bottle or by adding a drop to a tissue when you need a quick mental boost.

4. Blending: Create custom blends of essential oils to suit your preferences and specific focus needs.

Creating a Focus and Concentration Routine:

- Establish a dedicated study or work area where you practice aromatherapy consistently.

- Experiment with different essential oils to find the scents that resonate best with you for enhancing focus.

- Practice mindfulness while inhaling the scents, focusing on your tasks with intention.

Conclusion: Elevate Your Focus Naturally with Aromatherapy

Enhancing focus and concentration during study and work is attainable through the power of aromatherapy and essential oils. By incorporating these natural remedies into your routine, you can create a productive and energizing environment that supports mental clarity and cognitive performance. Remember that aromatherapy is a complementary approach, and it can be integrated into various aspects of your daily life to help you excel in your academic and professional endeavors. With the scents of nature by your side, you can navigate the challenges of focus and concentration with clarity and confidence.

Ancient Egyptian Essential Oil Recipes and Uses

Introduction:

The ancient Egyptians, known for their rich history and profound contributions to various fields, including medicine and cosmetics, were early pioneers in the use of essential oils for health, beauty, and spiritual purposes. Essential oils played a significant role in their daily lives, rituals, and healing practices. In this detailed text, we will delve into the world of ancient Egyptian essential oil recipes and their multifaceted uses, providing insight into the fascinating history and cultural significance of aromatic oils in ancient Egypt.

The Historical Significance of Essential Oils in Ancient Egypt:

The ancient Egyptians revered essential oils for their therapeutic, cosmetic, and spiritual properties. They believed that these aromatic substances held the power to connect the physical and spiritual realms and that they could enhance one's well-being and bridge the gap between the living and the divine.

Essential Oil Extraction in Ancient Egypt:

The process of extracting essential oils in ancient Egypt was labor-intensive and required specialized knowledge. Some of the methods employed included:

1. Infusion: Infusing aromatic plants in oils or fats to extract their scents and medicinal properties.

2. Distillation: The Egyptians were early adopters of distillation methods to extract essential oils from aromatic herbs and resins.

Ancient Egyptian Essential Oil Recipes and Uses:

1. Kyphi: Kyphi was a sacred incense and perfume made from a complex blend of aromatic ingredients, including frankincense, myrrh, honey, and wine. It was used in religious ceremonies and as a symbol of purification and connection to the divine.

2. Cosmetics: Essential oils, such as myrrh and cedarwood, were added to cosmetics, perfumes, and oils used for skincare, enhancing beauty and promoting radiant skin.

3. Healing Balms: Egyptians used essential oils to create healing balms and ointments for various ailments, including respiratory issues, wounds, and skin conditions.

4. Aromatherapy: Aromatherapy played a vital role in Egyptian medicine, where essential oils were inhaled or applied topically to alleviate physical and emotional imbalances.

5. Embalming: Myrrh and frankincense essential oils were prominent components of the embalming process, preserving the bodies of the deceased.

Practical Applications of Ancient Egyptian Essential Oils:

- Incorporate ancient Egyptian-inspired essential oil blends into your modern aromatherapy practices to connect with the wisdom of the past.

- Explore the use of essential oils in skincare and cosmetics, creating natural products reminiscent of those used by ancient Egyptians.

- Embrace the spiritual and meditative aspects of essential oils in your daily rituals, drawing inspiration from the ancient Egyptians' reverence for aromatic scents.

Conclusion: Honoring Tradition and Wisdom

The ancient Egyptians' profound knowledge of essential oils and their multifaceted uses continue to inspire us today. By exploring the recipes and practices of this ancient civilization, we can connect with the rich history and cultural significance of aromatic oils. Whether used for health, beauty, or spiritual purposes, essential oils remain a timeless and powerful tool for enhancing well-being and connecting with the wisdom of the past. As we embrace the legacy of ancient Egyptian aromatherapy, we honor a tradition that has shaped the world of essential oils and continues to impact our lives in meaningful ways.

Harnessing the Power of Resin Essential Oils: Myrrh, Frankincense, and Benzoin

Introduction:

Resin essential oils, derived from the sap or resin of trees, have been treasured for centuries for their therapeutic, spiritual, and aromatic properties. Among the most revered resin oils are myrrh, frankincense, and benzoin. These oils have played essential roles in various cultures and civilizations, from ancient rituals to modern holistic practices. In this detailed text, we will explore the fascinating world of resin essential oils, delving into the history, extraction methods, and versatile uses of myrrh, frankincense, and benzoin.

The Rich History of Resin Essential Oils:

Resin essential oils have been valued for thousands of years for their sacred and healing properties. They were used in religious ceremonies, as offerings to deities, and for medicinal purposes in ancient civilizations, including Egypt, India, and the Middle East.

Extraction Methods:

1. Myrrh (Commiphora myrrha): Myrrh essential oil is extracted from the resin of the myrrh tree through steam distillation. The resin is

harvested by making small cuts in the bark, allowing the sap to ooze out and harden.

2. Frankincense (Boswellia sacra): Frankincense essential oil is also obtained through steam distillation from the resin of the frankincense tree. The trees are carefully scored, and the resin is collected and processed into oil.

3. Benzoin (Styrax benzoin): Benzoin essential oil is derived from the resin of the benzoin tree. Unlike myrrh and frankincense, benzoin is extracted through solvent extraction or resinoid extraction, creating a thick, aromatic resinoid.

Therapeutic Benefits of Resin Essential Oils:

1. Myrrh:

- Antiseptic and wound-healing properties
- Emotional support and grounding
- Promotes healthy skin and oral hygiene

2. Frankincense:

- Reduces stress and anxiety
- Supports respiratory health
- Anti-inflammatory and analgesic effects

- Enhances spiritual and meditative practices

3. Benzoin:

- Eases respiratory congestion
- Provides emotional comfort and relaxation
- Supports skin health and regeneration

Versatile Uses of Resin Essential Oils:

1. Aromatherapy: Diffuse myrrh, frankincense, or benzoin essential oils to create a tranquil and sacred atmosphere for meditation and relaxation.

2. Topical Application: Dilute resin essential oils in a carrier oil for massage or apply them to pulse points for emotional support and skin health.

3. Skincare: Incorporate these oils into your skincare routine to promote healthy, youthful skin, reduce the appearance of scars, and soothe irritation.

4. Respiratory Support: Inhale vapor containing resin oils or add them to a steam inhalation for respiratory relief and clear breathing.

5. Spiritual and Ritual Use: Resin essential oils have a long history of use in spiritual and ritual practices, enhancing prayer, meditation, and sacred ceremonies.

Conclusion: Resin Essential Oils for Holistic Well-Being

Myrrh, frankincense, and benzoin essential oils, with their rich histories and therapeutic properties, continue to play essential roles in holistic well-being. Whether used for emotional support, physical healing, or spiritual enrichment, these resin essential oils offer a powerful connection to ancient traditions and a path to greater balance and harmony in our modern lives. As we harness the power of these sacred oils, we honor the wisdom of our ancestors and discover the profound benefits they bring to our holistic health and spiritual journey.

Essential Oils for Spiritual Protection and Cleansing

Introduction:

Throughout history, essential oils have been revered for their potent spiritual properties. These aromatic elixirs have been used for spiritual protection, purification, and energy cleansing in various cultures and belief systems. Whether you're seeking to create a sacred space, clear negative energy, or enhance your spiritual practice, essential oils can be powerful allies. In this detailed text, we'll explore the world of essential oils for spiritual protection and cleansing, delving into their history, significance, and practical applications.

The Significance of Spiritual Protection and Cleansing:

Spiritual protection and cleansing are practices that aim to create a harmonious and energetically balanced environment. They are essential in many spiritual and religious traditions to ward off negative energies, remove spiritual impurities, and invite positive vibrations.

Essential Oils for Spiritual Protection and Cleansing:

1. White Sage (Salvia apiana): White sage essential oil is renowned for its purifying properties. It's commonly used in smudging rituals to cleanse spaces of negative energy.

2. Cedarwood (Cedrus atlantica): Cedarwood essential oil has a grounding and protective energy. It's used to create a shield of spiritual protection.

3. Frankincense (Boswellia carterii): Frankincense essential oil is associated with elevated spiritual consciousness and purification. It's used in various religious ceremonies.

4. Myrrh (Commiphora myrrha): Myrrh essential oil is considered purifying and is often used to cleanse spaces and promote spiritual awareness.

5. Juniper Berry (Juniperus communis): Juniper berry essential oil has protective qualities and is used to banish negative energy.

Practical Applications:

1. Space Clearing: Create a spiritual protection spray by blending essential oils with water in a spray bottle. Use it to clear negative energy from your home or sacred space.

2. Anointing: Dilute essential oils in a carrier oil and use them to anoint yourself or objects during rituals and meditation.

3. Diffusion: Diffuse protective and cleansing essential oils in your space to maintain a spiritually pure environment.

4. Bath Rituals: Add a few drops of essential oil to your bath for personal purification and relaxation.

5. Crystal Charging: Place your crystals and gemstones with protective essential oils to cleanse and charge their energy.

Creating a Spiritual Protection Ritual:

- Begin with a clear intention for your protection or cleansing ritual.
- Choose the essential oils that resonate with your spiritual goals and needs.
- Use visualization and mindfulness to infuse your space or self with positive energy.
- Express gratitude and positive affirmations as you work with the oils.

Conclusion: Elevating Your Spiritual Journey

Essential oils are potent tools for enhancing your spiritual journey by providing protection and cleansing. Whether you're creating a sacred space, performing energy clearing, or deepening your spiritual practice, these oils can serve as powerful allies. As you incorporate essential oils into your spiritual rituals, you not only embrace ancient traditions but also elevate your spiritual journey to new heights. With intention and the energy of nature's essences, you can create a sanctuary of protection, purity, and spiritual enlightenment in your life.

Using Essential Oils to Support Recovery After Exercise

Introduction:

Exercise is essential for maintaining physical health, but the recovery process is equally important. Proper recovery allows your body to repair and rebuild, reducing the risk of injury and enhancing overall performance. Essential oils, with their natural properties, can be valuable allies in the -workout recovery journey. In this detailed text, we will explore the benefits of using essential oils to support recovery after exercise, including their applications, key oils, and practical tips for a holistic approach to -exercise well-being.

The Importance of -Exercise Recovery:

-exercise recovery is crucial for several reasons:

- Muscle Repair: After intense exercise, your muscles need time to repair microtears and grow stronger.

- Inflammation Control: Exercise can lead to inflammation, and proper recovery helps reduce inflammation and soreness.

- Injury Prevention: Adequate recovery minimizes the risk of overuse injuries caused by repetitive movements.

- Optimal Performance: Effective recovery ensures that you're ready for your next workout or physical activity.

Essential Oils for -Exercise Recovery:

1. Lavender (Lavandula angustifolia): Lavender essential oil is known for its soothing and anti-inflammatory properties. It can help reduce muscle soreness and promote relaxation.

2. Peppermint (Mentha × piperita): Peppermint oil has a cooling effect and can alleviate muscle discomfort. It's also energizing, making it useful for -workout fatigue.

3. Eucalyptus (Eucalyptus globulus): Eucalyptus essential oil can open the airways, making it helpful for respiratory support after exercise. It also has anti-inflammatory properties.

4. Arnica (Arnica montana): Arnica oil, derived from the arnica plant, is often used topically to reduce muscle pain and bruising.

5. Rosemary (Rosmarinus officinalis): Rosemary essential oil can improve circulation and relieve muscle tension when used in massage.

Practical Applications:

1. Massage: Dilute essential oils in a carrier oil and use them for a -workout massage to relax muscles and improve circulation.

2. Bath: Add a few drops of essential oil to a warm bath to soothe sore muscles and promote relaxation.

3. Compress: Create a hot or cold compress by adding essential oils to warm or cold water, then soaking a cloth and applying it to the affected area.

4. Inhalation: Inhale the aromatic scents of essential oils directly from the bottle or by adding a drop to a tissue for an instant energy boost.

5. Aromatherapy: Diffuse essential oils in your space to create a calming and recovery-enhancing atmosphere.

Holistic -Exercise Recovery Tips:

- Stay hydrated to support your body's natural detoxification processes.
- Incorporate stretching and yoga into your routine to improve flexibility and reduce muscle tension.
- Prioritize sleep to allow your body to repair and regenerate.

- Consider nutritional support with balanced -workout meals and supplements like protein and omega-3 fatty acids.

Conclusion: Enhancing Recovery Naturally

Recovery after exercise is vital for your overall health and fitness journey. Essential oils can be invaluable tools for promoting relaxation, reducing muscle soreness, and enhancing your -exercise recovery routine. By incorporating these natural remedies into your recovery plan, you can achieve a more holistic and balanced approach to fitness, supporting your body's natural healing processes and ensuring you're ready for your next workout with vitality and enthusiasm.

The Role of Essential Oils in Massage Therapy

Introduction:

Massage therapy has been practiced for centuries to promote relaxation, relieve pain, and enhance overall well-being. When combined with the therapeutic properties of essential oils, massage therapy becomes an even more potent tool for achieving physical and emotional balance. In this detailed text, we will explore the symbiotic relationship between essential oils and massage therapy, delving into the benefits, techniques, and key oils that can elevate your massage experience.

The Synergy of Essential Oils and Massage Therapy:

The integration of essential oils into massage therapy is known as aromatherapy massage. It combines the therapeutic benefits of touch and scent to create a holistic healing experience. Essential oils, extracted from aromatic plants, offer a wide range of physical and emotional benefits that complement the hands-on approach of massage.

Benefits of Aromatherapy Massage:

1. Relaxation: Aromatherapy massage induces a deep sense of relaxation, reducing stress and anxiety.

2. Pain Relief: Certain essential oils have analgesic properties that can alleviate muscle tension and reduce pain.

3. Improved Circulation: The combination of massage and essential oils can enhance blood circulation, promoting oxygen and nutrient delivery to tissues.

4. Emotional Balance: Aromatherapy can have a profound impact on mood and emotions, helping to uplift spirits or create a sense of calm.

5. Skin Benefits: Essential oils can nourish and rejuvenate the skin, making it an excellent addition to cosmetic massage treatments.

Key Essential Oils for Massage Therapy:

1. Lavender (Lavandula angustifolia): Lavender oil is renowned for its calming and soothing properties, making it a popular choice for relaxation massages.

2. Peppermint (Mentha × piperita): Peppermint oil's cooling sensation can relieve muscle tension and headaches during massage.

3. Eucalyptus (Eucalyptus globulus): Eucalyptus oil is used for respiratory massages, as it can open airways and ease congestion.

4. Chamomile (Matricaria chamomilla): Chamomile oil is excellent for sensitive skin and relaxation massages.

5. Rosemary (Rosmarinus officinalis): Rosemary oil can invigorate and energize during sports massages.

Aromatherapy Massage Techniques:

1. Effleurage: Long, sweeping strokes to warm up the muscles and distribute essential oils evenly.

2. Petrissage: Kneading and squeezing motions to release muscle tension.

3. Friction: Circular motions with fingers or thumbs to target specific areas.

4. Tapotement: Rhythmic tapping or percussion to stimulate circulation and invigorate muscles.

5. Stretching: Incorporating stretches into the massage to improve flexibility and range of motion.

Safety Precautions:

- Always dilute essential oils in a carrier oil to avoid skin irritation.
- Check for any allergies or sensitivities to specific oils.
- Communicate openly with your massage therapist about your preferences and any health concerns.

Conclusion: A Holistic Journey of Healing

Aromatherapy massage combines the art of touch with the science of scent, creating a holistic journey of healing and relaxation. Whether you seek relief from physical tension or emotional stress, the integration of essential oils into massage therapy can enhance your overall well-being. By working with trained therapists and selecting the right oils for your needs, you can experience the rejuvenating and transformative power of this ancient practice, leaving you with a profound sense of balance and vitality.

Olfaction and Memory: How Scents Trigger Recall

Introduction:

Our sense of smell, or olfaction, is a powerful and often underrated tool that plays a significant role in our everyday experiences. Beyond its role in identifying and enjoying aromas, our sense of smell has a remarkable connection to memory and emotion. In this detailed text, we will explore the fascinating relationship between olfaction and memory, delving into the science behind scent-triggered recall and its implications for our lives.

The Intricate Connection Between Smell and Memory:

The olfactory system, which includes the olfactory bulb and the brain's limbic system, is closely linked to memory and emotion. Unlike our other senses, smell is processed in these brain regions before being sent to the neocortex, where conscious perception occurs. This unique pathway allows scents to have a direct and profound impact on our memories and emotions.

How Scents Trigger Recall:

1. Associative Learning: When we encounter a particular scent while experiencing an event or emotion, our brain forms an association

between the scent and that memory. This association can lead to the recall of that memory when we encounter the same scent in the future.

2. Emotional Connection: Scents are powerful triggers of emotions. A familiar scent can evoke feelings associated with past experiences, whether they are joyful, nostalgic, or even melancholic.

3. Neurological Pathways: The olfactory bulb has direct connections to brain regions involved in memory and emotion, such as the amygdala and hippocampus. This direct wiring allows for rapid and strong memory recall.

The Proustian Phenomenon:

The famous writer Marcel Proust coined the term "Proustian phenomenon" to describe the powerful way in which a scent can transport us back in time through memory recall. In his novel "In Search of Lost Time," Proust's narrator dips a madeleine cookie into tea, and the scent and taste trigger a flood of childhood memories.

Practical Implications:

1. Aromatherapy: Aromatherapy utilizes the power of scents to influence emotions and well-being. Certain essential oils can promote relaxation, reduce anxiety, or enhance focus through their olfactory effects.

2. Personal and Cultural Significance: Scents often hold personal or cultural significance. Perfumes, spices, and foods are examples of scents that carry cultural and familial memories.

3. Therapeutic Uses: In therapeutic settings, the connection between smell and memory can be harnessed to help individuals with conditions like dementia or PTSD.

Conclusion: The Evocative Magic of Scents

The connection between olfaction and memory is a testament to the intricate workings of our brain. Scents have the remarkable ability to transport us through time and evoke vivid memories and emotions. Understanding this relationship allows us to appreciate the profound impact that scents can have on our lives, whether through the use of aromatherapy, the enjoyment of nostalgic fragrances, or the therapeutic potential for those in need. As we explore the world of scents and memories, we gain a deeper appreciation for the rich tapestry of our sensory experiences and the extraordinary capabilities of our brain.

Marjoram Essential Oil: A Versatile Oil for Health and Cooking

Introduction:

Marjoram essential oil, derived from the aromatic herb Origanum majorana, is a versatile and underrated oil that offers a wide range of health benefits and culinary delights. Known for its warm, herbaceous aroma, marjoram oil has been treasured for centuries for its therapeutic properties and its ability to enhance the flavor of various dishes. In this detailed text, we will explore the uses, benefits, and culinary applications of marjoram essential oil, shedding light on the many ways it can enhance your life.

The Essence of Marjoram:

Marjoram, also known as "joy of the mountains" in Greek, has a long history of use in traditional medicine and cuisine. The herb is native to the Mediterranean region and has a delightful fragrance that blends well with a variety of other oils and foods.

Therapeutic Benefits of Marjoram Essential Oil:

1. Relaxation and Stress Relief: Marjoram oil has calming properties that can help reduce stress and anxiety when diffused or applied topically.

2. Pain and Muscle Relief: It can be used in massage to alleviate muscle tension, ease joint discomfort, and promote relaxation.

3. Respiratory Support: Marjoram oil may aid in opening airways and promoting clear breathing when inhaled or used in steam inhalation.

4. Digestive Aid: When diluted and applied topically, it may help soothe digestive discomfort and support healthy digestion.

Culinary Applications of Marjoram Essential Oil:

1. Flavor Enhancer: Marjoram oil's warm and slightly sweet flavor makes it an excellent addition to a variety of dishes, including soups, stews, sauces, and roasted meats.

2. Salad Dressings: A drop or two of marjoram oil can elevate the taste of homemade salad dressings, lending a unique and savory note.

3. Baking: Incorporate marjoram oil into your bread, pizza dough, or focaccia recipes for an extra burst of flavor.

4. Marinades: Add marjoram oil to marinades for poultry, fish, or vegetables to infuse them with a delicious aroma and taste.

How to Use Marjoram Essential Oil:

1. Aromatherapy: Diffuse marjoram oil to create a calming and soothing atmosphere in your home.

2. Topical Application: Dilute marjoram oil with a carrier oil and apply it to the skin for massage or targeted relief.

3. Inhalation: Inhale the scent directly from the bottle or add a drop to a tissue for relaxation or respiratory support.

4. Cooking: Ensure that you use a food-grade marjoram essential oil and follow recommended usage guidelines for culinary applications.

Safety Precautions:

- Always dilute marjoram essential oil before applying it to the skin to avoid irritation.
- Consult with a healthcare professional, especially if you are pregnant, nursing, or taking medication.

Conclusion: Embrace the Versatility of Marjoram

Marjoram essential oil is a true gem in the world of essential oils, offering a delightful blend of therapeutic benefits and culinary versatility. Whether you seek relaxation, muscle relief, or a culinary adventure, marjoram oil can be a valuable addition to your wellness and kitchen arsenal. As you explore the many ways to incorporate marjoram oil into your daily life, you'll discover its unique ability to enhance both your physical well-being and your culinary creations, making it a cherished companion on your journey to health and flavorful cooking.

Crafting Scented Essential Oil Candles at Home

Introduction:

There's something magical about the warm glow and aromatic embrace of a scented candle. If you're a fan of both aromatherapy and crafting, why not combine the two and create your own scented essential oil candles at home? Making candles from scratch allows you to customize their scents and design, creating a personalized ambiance for your space. In this detailed text, we'll guide you through the art of crafting scented essential oil candles, from choosing the right materials to mastering the process.

Materials You'll Need:

1. Wax: Choose from paraffin wax, soy wax, or beeswax, depending on your preferences and availability.

2. Wick: Select a wick appropriate for your candle size and type of wax.

3. Fragrance: Essential oils of your choice for scenting the candles.

4. Colorant (Optional): If you want to add color to your candles, opt for candle dye or crayon shavings.

5. Double Boiler: To melt the wax safely.

6. Thermometer: To monitor the wax temperature.

7. Candle Molds or Containers: Choose from various shapes and sizes.

8. Stirring Utensil: A dedicated tool for stirring the wax and fragrance.

Steps to Crafting Scented Essential Oil Candles:

1. Prepare Your Workspace:

- Cover your work area with newspaper or a drop cloth to catch any wax drips.
- Set up your double boiler and have all materials within reach.

2. Measure and Cut the Wick:

- Cut the wick to the desired length, leaving a bit extra to account for securing it to the container or mold.

3. Melt the Wax:

- Place your chosen wax into the double boiler and heat it slowly until it's completely melted. Use a thermometer to monitor the temperature; most waxes melt between 160°F and 180°F (71°C to 82°C).

4. Add Fragrance:

- Once the wax is melted, remove it from heat and allow it to cool slightly. This is crucial to prevent the essential oils from evaporating.

- Add your chosen essential oils to the wax, stirring gently to ensure even distribution. The number of drops will depend on the volume of wax and your desired fragrance strength; typically, 10-15 drops per cup of wax is a good starting point.

5. Add Color (Optional):

- If you want colored candles, add the candle dye or crayon shavings to the wax and stir until it's evenly blended.

6. Secure the Wick:

- Dip the end of the wick into the melted wax and then press it into the center of the container or mold. This will secure the wick in place.

7. Pour the Wax:

- Carefully pour the scented and colored wax into your chosen container or mold.

8. Allow to Cool and Set:

- Let the candles cool and solidify completely. This may take a few hours.

9. Trim the Wick:

- Once the candles are fully set, trim the wick to your desired length, leaving about ¼ inch (0.6 cm) above the candle surface.

10. Enjoy Your Homemade Candles:

- Light your scented essential oil candles and bask in the delightful aroma and warm ambiance they create.

Safety Tips:

- Always follow safety guidelines when working with hot wax and open flames.
- Use essential oils that are safe for topical use and candle making.

- Keep candles away from flammable materials and never leave them unattended.

Conclusion: Personalized Aromatherapy

Crafting scented essential oil candles at home allows you to infuse your space with the scents that resonate with you most. Whether you're looking to create a calming oasis, a revitalizing atmosphere, or a cozy setting, homemade candles offer endless possibilities. This creative and therapeutic endeavor allows you to indulge in the art of candle making while enjoying the benefits of aromatherapy, making your space truly unique and inviting. So, gather your materials, let your creativity flow, and embrace the joy of crafting your very own scented candles.

Essential Oils for Menstrual Health: Alleviating Cramps and PMS

Introduction:

Menstruation is a natural part of a woman's life, but it often comes with discomfort and bothersome symptoms like menstrual cramps and premenstrual syndrome (PMS). While there are various methods to manage these issues, essential oils offer a natural and holistic approach to alleviating menstrual discomfort. In this detailed text, we will explore the benefits of using essential oils for menstrual health, focusing on how they can effectively reduce cramps and ease PMS symptoms.

Understanding Menstrual Cramps and PMS:

1. Menstrual Cramps: Menstrual cramps, also known as dysmenorrhea, are sharp or throbbing pains in the lower abdomen that occur before or during menstruation. They are caused by the contraction of the uterine muscles as they expel the uterine lining.

2. Premenstrual Syndrome (PMS): PMS encompasses a range of physical and emotional symptoms that occur in the days leading up to menstruation. These symptoms can include mood swings, bloating, breast tenderness, and irritability.

How Essential Oils Can Help:

Essential oils offer a natural and aromatherapeutic approach to managing menstrual discomfort. They can:

1. Relieve Muscle Tension: Certain essential oils have analgesic and muscle-relaxing properties that can ease the uterine muscle contractions responsible for cramps.

2. Balance Hormones: Some essential oils can help regulate hormonal fluctuations, reducing the severity of PMS symptoms.

3. Promote Relaxation: The calming and soothing scents of essential oils can alleviate stress and anxiety associated with menstruation.

Essential Oils for Menstrual Cramps:

1. Lavender (Lavandula angustifolia): Lavender oil has calming properties that can help reduce pain and muscle tension.

2. Clary Sage (Salvia sclarea): Clary sage oil is known for its ability to relieve muscle cramps and balance hormones.

3. Peppermint (Mentha × piperita): Peppermint oil's cooling sensation can provide relief from cramps when applied topically.

4. Roman Chamomile (Chamaemelum nobile): Chamomile oil has anti-inflammatory properties that can help ease cramp-related inflammation.

Essential Oils for PMS:

1. Geranium (Pelargonium graveolens): Geranium oil can help balance hormones and reduce mood swings associated with PMS.

2. Ylang Ylang (Cananga odorata): Ylang ylang oil is known for its mood-enhancing properties and can help alleviate PMS-related stress.

3. Bergamot (Citrus bergamia): Bergamot oil can uplift the mood and reduce feelings of irritability and tension.

Ways to Use Essential Oils:

1. Topical Application: Dilute essential oils with a carrier oil and apply them to the abdomen for targeted relief. Massage gently in a circular motion.

2. Aromatherapy: Diffuse essential oils in your space to create a calming atmosphere. Inhaling the scents can help reduce stress and discomfort.

3. Warm Baths: Add a few drops of essential oil to a warm bath to relax muscles and ease tension.

Safety Considerations:

- Always dilute essential oils with a carrier oil before applying them to the skin to avoid irritation.
- Perform a patch test to check for any allergic reactions before using a new essential oil.
- Consult with a healthcare professional if you have underlying health conditions or are pregnant.

Conclusion: Natural Relief for Menstrual Discomfort

Essential oils provide a natural and holistic approach to managing menstrual cramps and PMS symptoms. By incorporating these aromatic remedies into your menstrual care routine, you can find relief from discomfort, experience emotional balance, and make your monthly cycle a more manageable and enjoyable experience. Remember to choose essential oils that resonate with you personally and seek professional advice if you have specific concerns or conditions. With the soothing power of essential oils, you can embrace your menstrual health with greater ease and comfort.

The Art of Blending Perfumes: Combining Notes for Unique Scents

Introduction:

Perfume is a timeless and personal accessory that has the power to evoke emotions, memories, and a sense of identity. While many exquisite perfumes are available on the market, there's a unique pleasure in creating your own custom fragrance. The art of blending perfumes allows you to craft scents that reflect your personality and style. In this detailed text, we will delve into the fascinating world of perfume blending, exploring how to combine fragrance notes to create a truly unique and signature scent.

Understanding Fragrance Notes:

1. Top Notes: These are the initial scents that you detect when you first apply a fragrance. Top notes are often fresh and light, designed to grab your attention but evaporate relatively quickly.

2. Middle Notes (Heart Notes): Middle notes emerge after the top notes have faded. They provide the body and character of the fragrance and are often floral or fruity.

3. Base Notes: Base notes are the foundation of the fragrance, providing depth and longevity. They are typically rich, woody, or musky scents that linger on the skin for hours.

Steps to Blending Perfumes:

1. Gather Your Materials:

- Essential oils or fragrance oils of your choice.
- Blotter strips or testing strips.
- A small glass or plastic perfume bottle.
- A notebook to record your formulations.

2. Choose Your Fragrance Family:

- Perfume fragrances are categorized into families such as floral, oriental, citrus, and woody. Decide which family you'd like to explore.

3. Select Your Key Notes:

- Start by choosing a few essential oils or fragrance oils that will serve as the core of your blend. These will be your top, middle, and base notes.

4. Experiment with Blotter Strips:

- Apply a drop of each chosen oil onto separate blotter strips. Smell and note how they interact. Pay attention to how they evolve over time.

5. Create a Formula:

- Decide on the ratio of top, middle, and base notes in your perfume. For example, a common formula is 30% top notes, 50% middle notes, and 20% base notes.

6. Blend and Test:

- Carefully blend your chosen oils in a small glass or plastic perfume bottle. Start with a small batch to experiment.

- Allow the blend to mature for at least a week to let the notes meld and evolve.

- Test the perfume on your skin, as your body chemistry can alter the scent.

7. Refine Your Blend:

- Take notes on your impressions and any adjustments needed. You may need to tweak the ratios or add new notes to achieve the desired scent.

8. Finalize Your Perfume:

- Once you're satisfied with your blend, transfer it into a beautiful perfume bottle for storage and daily use.

Tips for Perfume Blending:

- Use a dropper for precise measurements.
- Don't rush the blending process; patience is key.
- Experiment with different combinations and ratios.
- Keep a journal to record your formulations and results.
- Use high-quality oils for the best results.

Conclusion: Craft Your Signature Scent

Blending perfumes is an art form that allows you to express your individuality and create scents that resonate with your unique style. Whether you prefer floral, oriental, citrus, or woody fragrances, the possibilities are endless. With a little experimentation, creativity, and patience, you can craft your signature scent that reflects your personality and leaves a lasting impression. Embrace the art of perfume blending and embark on a fragrant journey to create scents that are uniquely and beautifully yours.

Safely Incorporating Essential Oils into Your Skincare Routine

Introduction:

The world of skincare is ever-evolving, with an increasing emphasis on natural and holistic approaches. Essential oils, derived from plants, have gained popularity for their potential benefits in skincare. However, it's essential to use them safely and effectively to reap the rewards without risking skin irritation or other adverse reactions. In this detailed text, we'll explore the safe incorporation of essential oils into your skincare routine, providing you with valuable insights and guidelines.

Understanding Essential Oils:

1. Essential Oils Basics: Essential oils are highly concentrated extracts from plants, flowers, leaves, or fruits. They contain the essence and aroma of the plant and are used in skincare for their potential therapeutic properties.

2. Dilution: Due to their potency, essential oils must be diluted before applying to the skin. Carrier oils like jojoba, coconut, or almond oil are often used for this purpose.

Choosing the Right Essential Oils:

1. Skin Type: Consider your skin type and specific concerns when selecting essential oils. For example, lavender and chamomile are gentle and suitable for most skin types, while tea tree oil is beneficial for acne-prone skin.

2. Quality Matters: Invest in high-quality, pure essential oils from reputable brands to ensure they are free from additives or contaminants.

Safe Incorporation into Your Skincare Routine:

1. Patch Test: Before using any essential oil on your face, conduct a patch test on a small area of skin to check for allergies or irritation. Wait 24 hours to see if there's a reaction.

2. Dilution Ratios: Follow recommended dilution ratios, typically 1-2% for facial skincare. This means 1-2 drops of essential oil per 1 teaspoon of carrier oil.

3. Spot Treatments: For specific issues like blemishes, consider spot treatments with highly diluted essential oils.

4. Avoid Sun Exposure: Some essential oils, like citrus oils, can make your skin more sensitive to sunlight. Use caution and apply them in the evening or use sunscreen during the day.

5. Storage: Store essential oils in a cool, dark place away from direct sunlight to preserve their quality.

Essential Oils for Common Skin Concerns:

1. Acne: Tea tree, lavender, and chamomile oils have anti-inflammatory and antibacterial properties that can help with acne.

2. Dry Skin: Try essential oils like rose, geranium, or frankincense, which can help hydrate and soothe dry skin.

3. Oily Skin: Lemon, lemongrass, and cedarwood oils may help balance excess oil production.

4. Aging Skin: Rosehip seed oil and frankincense are often used to address signs of aging like fine lines and wrinkles.

DIY Essential Oil Recipes:

1. Hydrating Face Serum:

- 1 oz (30 ml) jojoba oil

- 4 drops rose essential oil
- 2 drops frankincense essential oil
- 2 drops lavender essential oil

2. Acne Spot Treatment:

- 1 tsp aloe vera gel
- 1 drop tea tree essential oil
- 1 drop lavender essential oil

Conclusion: Nourish Your Skin Naturally

Incorporating essential oils into your skincare routine can be a delightful and effective way to address various skin concerns. However, safety should always be a priority. By following proper dilution guidelines, conducting patch tests, and choosing essential oils that suit your skin type, you can harness the power of nature to nourish and enhance your skin safely. Embrace the world of essential oils in skincare, and enjoy the natural beauty benefits they offer for healthy and radiant skin.

Essential Oils for Travel: Staying Well on Your Journeys

Introduction:

Traveling is a wonderful adventure that allows us to explore new places and cultures. However, it often comes with its own set of challenges, including exposure to different environments, stress, and the risk of minor health issues. Essential oils can be valuable companions on your journeys, offering natural solutions to support your well-being while you explore the world. In this detailed text, we will explore the use of essential oils for travel, providing tips and remedies to help you stay well and enjoy your adventures to the fullest.

The Benefits of Essential Oils for Travel:

1. Portable Wellness: Essential oils are compact and easy to carry, making them ideal for travel.

2. Natural Remedies: Essential oils offer natural solutions for common travel-related issues like jet lag, motion sickness, and insect bites.

3. Emotional Support: They can help alleviate stress, anxiety, and sleep disturbances that may arise during travel.

Essential Oils for Common Travel Concerns:

1. Jet Lag: Peppermint, ginger, and citrus oils can help combat fatigue and promote alertness.

2. Motion Sickness: Ginger and peppermint oils can ease nausea and discomfort.

3. Stress and Anxiety: Lavender, chamomile, and bergamot oils are calming and can reduce travel-related stress.

4. Sleep Difficulties: Lavender, cedarwood, and frankincense oils can promote restful sleep in unfamiliar environments.

5. Insect Repellent: Citronella, eucalyptus, and lemongrass oils can help keep pesky insects at bay.

Travel-Friendly Essential Oil Remedies:

1. Jet Lag Roll-On:

- 10 ml roller bottle
- 5 drops peppermint essential oil
- 3 drops lavender essential oil
- 2 drops lemon essential oil

- Fill with a carrier oil (e.g., jojoba or fractionated coconut oil)
- Apply to pulse points during travel and upon arrival.

2. Motion Sickness Inhaler:
   - Blank inhaler tube
   - 3 drops ginger essential oil
   - 3 drops peppermint essential oil
   - Inhale as needed during travel.

3. Stress Relief Diffuser Blend:
   - Diffuser
   - 3 drops lavender essential oil
   - 2 drops bergamot essential oil
   - 2 drops frankincense essential oil
   - Use in your accommodation to create a calming atmosphere.

Safety Tips for Traveling with Essential Oils:

1. Pack Carefully: Ensure your essential oils are securely sealed to prevent leaks in your luggage.

2. Compliance: Be aware of airline regulations regarding liquids and essential oils in carry-on luggage.

3. Dilution: Always dilute essential oils properly before applying them to the skin, especially when trying new blends.

4. Patch Test: Test a small amount of diluted oil on your skin before using it extensively, especially if you have sensitive skin.

Conclusion: Travel Well, Travel Happy

Traveling is a rewarding experience that allows us to explore and create lasting memories. By incorporating essential oils into your travel routine, you can address common travel concerns naturally and enhance your overall well-being while on the road. Whether you're combating jet lag, staying calm during stressful moments, or protecting yourself from insects, essential oils are versatile companions for your journeys. So, pack your oils, embark on your adventures, and enjoy every moment of your travel with a sense of well-being and vitality.

Aromatherapy for the Elderly: Enhancing Quality of Life

Introduction:

As we age, maintaining physical, mental, and emotional well-being becomes increasingly important. Aromatherapy, the practice of using essential oils to promote health and well-being, can be a valuable tool for enhancing the quality of life for the elderly. In this detailed text, we will explore the benefits of aromatherapy for the elderly and provide insights into how it can be safely and effectively integrated into their daily routines, promoting relaxation, improved mood, and overall well-being.

Benefits of Aromatherapy for the Elderly:

1. Emotional Well-Being: Aromatherapy can uplift moods, reduce anxiety, and alleviate symptoms of depression, which can be common among the elderly.

2. Cognitive Support: Certain essential oils can support cognitive function and memory, potentially benefiting those dealing with age-related cognitive decline.

3. Physical Comfort: Aromatherapy can help ease aches, pains, and discomfort associated with aging, such as arthritis or muscle stiffness.

4. Improved Sleep: Many essential oils promote relaxation and better sleep, which can be particularly beneficial for seniors who may struggle with sleep disorders.

Safe Practices for Aromatherapy with the Elderly:

1. Consultation: Before using essential oils, consult with a healthcare professional, especially if the elderly person has underlying health conditions or is taking medications.

2. Proper Dilution: Essential oils should be diluted with a carrier oil to avoid skin irritation. A common dilution ratio is 1-2% for the elderly.

3. Patch Testing: Perform a patch test to check for allergic reactions before using a new essential oil on the skin.

4. Inhalation: Inhalation methods, such as using a diffuser or inhaling from a tissue, are often safer and more suitable for the elderly than topical application.

5. Avoid Photosensitive Oils: Some essential oils, like citrus oils, can make the skin more sensitive to sunlight. Use caution and avoid sun exposure after using these oils topically.

Essential Oils for the Elderly:

1. Lavender (Lavandula angustifolia): Lavender oil is renowned for its calming properties and can promote relaxation and better sleep.

2. Frankincense (Boswellia serrata): Frankincense is often used for its potential cognitive support and mood-enhancing effects.

3. Peppermint (Mentha × piperita): Peppermint oil can help alleviate digestive discomfort and provide a refreshing scent.

4. Rosemary (Rosmarinus officinalis): Rosemary oil may support cognitive function and memory.

5. Chamomile (Chamaemelum nobile): Chamomile is soothing and can help reduce anxiety and improve sleep.

Practical Aromatherapy Ideas:

1. Aromatherapy Diffuser: Place a diffuser with a calming essential oil blend in the living area to create a peaceful atmosphere.

2. Massage: Dilute essential oils with a carrier oil and use for gentle massages to ease muscle discomfort.

3. Pillow Spray: Create a pillow spray with lavender oil to promote restful sleep.

4. Inhalation: Inhaling essential oils from a tissue or handkerchief can provide quick relief from stress or anxiety.

Conclusion: A Fragrant Path to Well-Being

Aromatherapy offers a gentle and holistic approach to enhancing the quality of life for the elderly. By incorporating the soothing scents of essential oils into their daily routines, we can support emotional well-being, cognitive function, and physical comfort. However, it's crucial to exercise caution and follow safe practices when using essential oils with seniors. With the right guidance and care, aromatherapy can be a valuable tool for promoting a sense of well-being, comfort, and relaxation among the elderly, enriching their lives in the golden years.

Essential Oils in the Bible: Anointing and Healing Practices

Introduction:

The use of essential oils has a rich history that dates back thousands of years, and it's fascinating to discover that their presence can be traced back to biblical times. Essential oils played a significant role in ancient cultures, including those described in the Bible. In this detailed text, we will explore the historical and spiritual significance of essential oils in the Bible, shedding light on their role in anointing rituals, healing practices, and daily life during ancient times.

Essential Oils in Biblical Context:

1. Extraction Methods: Essential oils mentioned in the Bible were often extracted through methods like steam distillation, enfleurage, and maceration, much like modern extraction techniques.

2. Ancient Healing: Essential oils were used for their therapeutic properties in ancient times to address various physical and emotional ailments.

3. Symbolism: In biblical narratives, essential oils are often symbolically associated with healing, purification, and spiritual renewal.

Notable Essential Oils in the Bible:

1. Frankincense: One of the most famous biblical essential oils, frankincense, was considered a sacred resin used in religious rituals and as a symbol of divinity. It was gifted to the infant Jesus by the Magi.

2. Myrrh: Myrrh, another sacred resin, was used in anointing oils and for embalming. It was also among the gifts presented to the baby Jesus.

3. Cassia: Cassia, similar to cinnamon, was used in anointing oils in the Bible. It is associated with holiness and righteousness.

4. Spikenard: Spikenard was a precious and costly oil used for anointing and perfuming. It is famously mentioned in the story of Mary anointing Jesus' feet.

5. Hyssop: Hyssop was used for purification rituals and symbolized spiritual cleansing.

Biblical References to Essential Oils:

1. Exodus 30:23-25: This passage describes the holy anointing oil, which includes myrrh, cinnamon, cassia, and other fragrant ingredients.

2. Song of Solomon 4:13-14: A poetic description of a garden mentions spices and essential oils like saffron, calamus, cinnamon, and frankincense.

3. Matthew 2:11: The Magi's gifts to the baby Jesus included gold, frankincense, and myrrh.

Healing and Anointing Practices:

1. Spiritual Anointing: Anointing with oil was a significant religious practice in the Bible. It symbolized consecration, healing, and the presence of the Holy Spirit.

2. Medicinal Use: Essential oils were used for their therapeutic properties in biblical times. They were applied to wounds, used for massage, and inhaled for their healing effects.

3. Perfumery: Fragrant oils like myrrh and spikenard were used in perfumery and personal care, enhancing one's physical and emotional well-being.

Conclusion: Aromatic Legacy

The use of essential oils in the Bible reveals a rich history deeply intertwined with spirituality, healing, and daily life in ancient times.

These precious oils held symbolic and practical significance, from anointing rituals to medicinal applications. Today, the legacy of essential oils continues, as we rediscover and embrace their therapeutic and aromatic qualities, connecting us to an ancient tradition of well-being and spiritual significance. The presence of essential oils in the Bible reminds us of their enduring value in enhancing our physical, emotional, and spiritual lives.

The Role of Aromatherapists in Holistic Healthcare

Introduction:

Aromatherapy, the practice of using essential oils for therapeutic purposes, has gained popularity in recent years as people seek holistic approaches to health and well-being. Aromatherapists, trained professionals in the field of aromatherapy, play a vital role in guiding individuals towards better physical and emotional health. In this detailed text, we will explore the multifaceted role of aromatherapists in holistic healthcare, shedding light on their skills, responsibilities, and the benefits they bring to individuals seeking natural and holistic solutions.

Understanding Aromatherapy:

1. Essential Oils: Aromatherapists work with essential oils, highly concentrated plant extracts known for their therapeutic properties.

2. Holistic Approach: Aromatherapy takes a holistic approach to health, considering physical, emotional, and mental well-being as interconnected aspects of a person's health.

The Role of Aromatherapists:

1. Assessment: Aromatherapists conduct thorough assessments of clients' physical and emotional health, considering their medical history, lifestyle, and specific concerns.

2. Customization: Based on assessments, aromatherapists create personalized aromatherapy plans, recommending specific essential oils and application methods tailored to each client's needs.

3. Essential Oil Blending: Aromatherapists are skilled in blending essential oils to create unique formulations that address specific health issues or promote overall well-being.

4. Application Techniques: They guide clients on safe and effective ways to use essential oils, including topical application, inhalation, and diffusion.

5. Education: Aromatherapists educate clients about the properties of essential oils, potential contraindications, and self-care practices that can support their health goals.

Benefits of Aromatherapy in Holistic Healthcare:

1. Stress Reduction: Aromatherapy can help reduce stress, anxiety, and promote relaxation, which are essential for overall well-being.

2. Pain Management: Aromatherapy can complement pain management strategies, offering relief from conditions like chronic pain and headaches.

3. Emotional Support: Essential oils can aid in managing emotions, supporting individuals dealing with issues like depression, grief, or trauma.

4. Improved Sleep: Aromatherapists often help clients with sleep disorders by recommending calming essential oils and relaxation techniques.

5. Enhanced Immunity: Some essential oils have immune-boosting properties, contributing to better overall health.

Training and Certification:

1. Formal Education: Aromatherapists typically undergo formal training programs that cover essential oil chemistry, safety, and application methods.

2. Certification: Many aromatherapists obtain certification from recognized organizations to ensure they meet high professional standards.

Collaboration in Holistic Healthcare:

1. Team Approach: Aromatherapists often collaborate with other healthcare professionals, such as naturopaths, massage therapists, and chiropractors, to provide integrated care.

2. Complementary Therapy: Aromatherapy can complement conventional medical treatments, offering additional support for patients.

Conclusion: Nurturing Health and Well-Being

Aromatherapists are essential guides on the journey to holistic health and well-being. Their expertise in essential oils, personalized approaches to wellness, and ability to address both physical and emotional health issues make them valuable assets in the field of holistic healthcare. As individuals seek natural and complementary therapies to support their health, aromatherapists stand ready to provide guidance and solutions that nurture the body, mind, and spirit, promoting a balanced and harmonious approach to well-being.

Floral Hydrosols: Gentle Aromatics for Sensitive Skin

Introduction:

When it comes to skincare, especially for those with sensitive or delicate skin, the search for gentle yet effective products can be a never-ending quest. Floral hydrosols, also known as floral waters or hydrolats, have emerged as a soothing and natural solution. These aromatic waters offer a myriad of benefits, from hydration to calming irritation, making them a perfect choice for sensitive skin. In this detailed article, we will explore what floral hydrosols are, their benefits, how to use them, and why they are a boon for those seeking gentle skincare.

What Are Floral Hydrosols?

Floral hydrosols are aromatic waters created through the steam distillation of plant materials, typically flowers, and other botanicals. They are the byproduct of essential oil production, capturing the water-soluble compounds of the plant along with a subtle, natural fragrance. Unlike essential oils, which are highly concentrated and need to be diluted, floral hydrosols are much gentler and can be used directly on the skin.

Benefits of Floral Hydrosols for Sensitive Skin:

1. Hydration: Floral hydrosols are excellent hydrators. They help replenish the skin's moisture barrier, reducing dryness and flakiness, common issues for sensitive skin.

2. Calming: Many floral hydrosols, such as rose and chamomile, have soothing and anti-inflammatory properties. They can help reduce redness and irritation.

3. Balancing: Floral waters can help balance the skin's pH levels, preventing excess oil production and breakouts without drying out the skin.

4. Anti-Aging: Some floral hydrosols are rich in antioxidants that combat free radicals, which can lead to premature aging. They support a youthful complexion.

5. Refreshing: A quick spritz of floral hydrosol can provide an instant refreshment, making them ideal for on-the-go hydration.

Popular Floral Hydrosols for Sensitive Skin:

1. Rose Hydrosol: Known for its luxurious scent, rose hydrosol is a favorite for sensitive skin. It's moisturizing, calming, and helps reduce redness.

2. Chamomile Hydrosol: Chamomile is renowned for its anti-inflammatory properties. Its hydrosol is gentle and ideal for soothing irritated skin.

3. Lavender Hydrosol: Lavender is a versatile hydrosol that offers both relaxation and skin benefits. It's calming, healing, and helps with acne-prone skin.

4. Calendula Hydrosol: Calendula is excellent for healing and reducing inflammation, making it perfect for sensitive and damaged skin.

How to Use Floral Hydrosols:

1. Toner: Apply floral hydrosol directly to clean skin as a toner. It helps balance the skin's pH and prepares it for serums or moisturizers.

2. Hydration Mist: Keep a small spray bottle of hydrosol in your bag to refresh and hydrate your skin throughout the day.

3. Makeup Setting Spray: Use a gentle floral hydrosol as a makeup setting spray for a natural and dewy finish.

4. Compress: Soak a clean cloth in cold or room-temperature hydrosol and use it as a compress to calm irritated skin.

5. Add to Masks: Mix hydrosol with clay masks or powdered exfoliants for a spa-like experience.

Conclusion: Nurturing Sensitive Skin Naturally

Floral hydrosols offer a natural and gentle approach to skincare, making them an ideal choice for those with sensitive skin. Their hydrating, calming, and balancing properties, coupled with their subtle natural fragrances, provide a delightful and effective skincare experience. Whether used as a toner, hydration mist, or in various DIY skincare recipes, floral hydrosols are a versatile addition to any sensitive skin care routine. Embrace the gentle power of these aromatic waters and discover the soothing benefits they can bring to your skin, allowing you to nurture and care for it naturally.

Essential Oils for Acne and Blemish Control: Nature's Answer to Clearer Skin

Introduction:

Acne, a common skin condition that affects people of all ages, can be a source of frustration and self-consciousness. While there are numerous skincare products available, many individuals are turning to natural remedies like essential oils to combat acne and achieve clearer, healthier skin. In this comprehensive article, we will explore the causes of acne, the science behind essential oils, and the best essential oils for acne and blemish control. Whether you're dealing with occasional breakouts or persistent acne, these natural solutions may be the key to achieving smoother, blemish-free skin.

Understanding Acne: Causes and Types

Acne occurs when hair follicles become clogged with oil and dead skin cells, leading to the formation of pimples, blackheads, whiteheads, and even cysts. Several factors contribute to acne, including hormonal fluctuations, excess sebum production, bacteria (Propionibacterium acnes), and inflammation. It's essential to recognize that acne can manifest in various forms:

1. Whiteheads: Closed, clogged pores with a white or flesh-colored bump.

2. Blackheads: Open, clogged pores with a black or darkened surface.

3. Papules: Small, red, tender bumps without a visible center.

4. Pustules: Red, swollen pimples with a white or yellow center.

5. Nodules: Large, painful, solid lumps beneath the skin's surface.

6. Cysts: Deep, painful, pus-filled lumps that can cause scarring.

How Essential Oils Can Help: The Science Behind It

Essential oils are highly concentrated extracts from plants, each with its own unique chemical composition. Many essential oils possess properties that make them effective in combating acne:

1. Anti-Inflammatory: Essential oils like lavender and chamomile can reduce redness and inflammation associated with acne.

2. Antibacterial: Oils like tea tree and thyme have antimicrobial properties that can help kill acne-causing bacteria.

3. Sebum Regulation: Some essential oils, such as rosemary and geranium, can help regulate sebum production, preventing clogged pores.

4. Skin Healing: Oils like frankincense and helichrysum promote skin healing and reduce the risk of scarring.

5. Antioxidant: Essential oils rich in antioxidants, like lavender and rose, combat free radicals that contribute to acne.

Best Essential Oils for Acne and Blemish Control:

1. Tea Tree Oil (Melaleuca alternifolia): Known for its potent antibacterial properties, tea tree oil can effectively target acne-causing bacteria.

2. Lavender Oil (Lavandula angustifolia): Lavender oil is anti-inflammatory and promotes skin healing, reducing the appearance of blemishes.

3. Chamomile Oil (Matricaria chamomilla): Chamomile's anti-inflammatory and calming properties soothe irritated skin.

4. Geranium Oil (Pelargonium graveolens): Geranium oil helps balance sebum production, making it suitable for oily and combination skin.

5. Frankincense Oil (Boswellia serrata): Frankincense promotes skin regeneration and reduces the risk of scarring.

6. Helichrysum Oil (Helichrysum italicum): Helichrysum's wound-healing properties can help fade acne scars.

How to Use Essential Oils for Acne:

1. Dilution: Essential oils are highly concentrated and should be diluted with a carrier oil, such as jojoba or coconut oil, before applying to the skin.

2. Spot Treatment: Apply diluted essential oils directly to blemishes using a cotton swab or clean fingertip.

3. Facial Steam: Add a few drops of essential oil to a bowl of hot water, create a tent with a towel, and steam your face to open pores.

4. Face Masks: Incorporate essential oils into DIY face masks or clay masks for acne-prone skin.

5. Cleansers and Toners: Mix a few drops of essential oil into your cleanser or toner for daily use.

6. Aromatherapy: Diffuse essential oils like tea tree or lavender in your living space to reduce stress, which can exacerbate acne.

Conclusion: A Natural Path to Clearer Skin

Essential oils offer a natural and effective approach to managing acne and achieving clearer skin. By understanding the causes of acne and the science behind essential oils, individuals can harness the power of these plant extracts to combat breakouts, reduce inflammation, and promote skin healing. Whether used as a spot treatment, in skincare products, or in aromatherapy, essential oils provide a gentle yet potent solution to the age-old quest for blemish-free, radiant skin. Embrace the natural path to clearer skin and unlock the transformative potential of essential oils in your skincare routine.

Understanding the Quality of Essential Oils: Purity and Grading

Introduction:

Essential oils have gained immense popularity for their therapeutic and aromatic properties. However, with the growing demand, the market has seen an influx of essential oils of varying quality. To make informed choices and maximize the benefits of essential oils, it's crucial to understand the concept of purity and grading. In this comprehensive article, we will delve into what makes essential oils pure, the grading systems used, and how to ensure you're purchasing high-quality essential oils for your well-being.

The Essence of Purity: What Makes an Essential Oil Pure?

Essential oils are extracted from plant materials using various methods, such as steam distillation, cold-press extraction, or solvent extraction. The purity of an essential oil depends on several factors:

1. Source: High-quality essential oils start with premium plant material. The species, variety, and geographic origin of the plants play a vital role in the oil's quality.

2. Extraction Method: The extraction process should preserve the delicate chemical constituents of the plant without introducing contaminants.

3. Purity: Pure essential oils should contain only the volatile aromatic compounds from the plant, without additives, synthetic fragrances, or dilution.

4. Testing: Reputable producers conduct rigorous testing to verify the oil's authenticity, purity, and chemical composition.

The Grading Systems: Understanding Essential Oil Grades

Essential oils are often categorized into different grades based on their quality, purity, and intended use. Two common grading systems are:

1. Therapeutic Grade: This term is often used by essential oil companies to imply a high level of purity and quality. However, it's essential to note that there is no universally accepted standard for "therapeutic grade." It's a marketing term rather than a regulated classification.

2. Certified Pure Therapeutic Grade (CPTG): This grade is specific to doTERRA essential oils. It emphasizes rigorous testing and quality control. While it may indicate a certain level of quality, it's essential to scrutinize the testing procedures used by each company.

Ensuring the Quality of Essential Oils: What to Look For

1. Botanical Name: Check that the essential oil's botanical name matches the plant species you intend to use. Small variations can significantly affect the oil's properties.

2. Testing: Reputable companies provide batch-specific testing results, including gas chromatography and mass spectrometry (GC/MS) reports. These tests confirm the oil's chemical composition and purity.

3. Transparency: Choose brands that are transparent about their sourcing and production methods. Look for companies that provide information about the plant's origin and the extraction process.

4. Bottle Integrity: Essential oils should be stored in dark glass bottles to protect them from light and air, which can degrade the oil's quality. Ensure the bottle is sealed and tamper-evident.

5. Price: High-quality essential oils typically come at a higher price due to the labor-intensive extraction process and sourcing of premium plant material. Be cautious of extremely low-priced oils, as they may be of lower quality.

6. Reputation: Research the reputation of the essential oil brand and read customer reviews. Recommendations from trusted sources can also be valuable.

Conclusion: Navigating the World of Essential Oils

Understanding the quality of essential oils is essential for harnessing their therapeutic benefits effectively. The concepts of purity and grading help consumers make informed choices in a market flooded with options. By examining the source, extraction method, testing procedures, and reputation of essential oil brands, individuals can confidently select oils that align with their wellness goals. Embrace the world of essential oils with knowledge and discernment, and experience the true essence of nature's aromatic treasures.

Aromatherapy for ADHD: Calming and Focusing Children

Introduction:

Attention Deficit Hyperactivity Disorder (ADHD) is a neurodevelopmental disorder that affects children and adults, impacting their ability to focus, control impulses, and manage hyperactivity. While medication and therapy are commonly used treatments, some individuals and parents seek complementary approaches like aromatherapy to support ADHD management. In this comprehensive article, we will explore the potential benefits of aromatherapy for ADHD, the best essential oils to use, and safe practices to help children find calm and focus.

Understanding ADHD: Challenges and Management

ADHD is characterized by a range of symptoms, including inattention, hyperactivity, and impulsivity. Managing ADHD often involves a multifaceted approach that may include behavioral therapy, medication, and lifestyle adjustments. Aromatherapy is considered a complementary approach that may offer support but should not replace evidence-based treatments.

Aromatherapy for ADHD: How It Works

Aromatherapy involves using the aromatic compounds of essential oils to influence mood and behavior. While research on aromatherapy for ADHD is limited, some essential oils may have properties that promote relaxation, improve focus, and reduce hyperactivity. The following essential oils have shown promise in supporting ADHD management:

1. Lavender (Lavandula angustifolia): Lavender oil is known for its calming and soothing effects. It may help reduce restlessness and promote relaxation.

2. Vetiver (Vetiveria zizanioides): Vetiver oil has grounding properties and may improve focus and concentration.

3. Cedarwood (Juniperus virginiana): Cedarwood oil may have a calming effect, reducing impulsivity and hyperactivity.

4. Frankincense (Boswellia serrata): Frankincense is believed to promote emotional balance and mental clarity, potentially helping with ADHD symptoms.

5. Roman Chamomile (Chamaemelum nobile): Chamomile oil may have a soothing effect on the nervous system, aiding in relaxation.

Safe Practices for Aromatherapy with Children:

When using aromatherapy for children, especially those with ADHD, safety is paramount:

1. Dilution: Always dilute essential oils with a carrier oil before applying to the skin. The general guideline is 1-3 drops of essential oil per ounce of carrier oil.

2. Patch Test: Perform a patch test on a small area of skin to check for any allergic reactions or skin sensitivities.

3. Diffusion: Use an essential oil diffuser to disperse the aroma into the air. Diffusion is a safe method for children, as long as the oil is well-diluted.

4. Inhalation: Aromatherapy inhalers or personal diffusers can be used as a portable and safe option for children.

5. Supervision: Always supervise children when using essential oils, and keep oils out of their reach.

6. Consultation: If your child has other medical conditions or takes medications, consult with a healthcare professional before using essential oils.

Aromatherapy as a Complementary Approach:

It's important to view aromatherapy as a complementary approach rather than a standalone treatment for ADHD. Aromatherapy can be integrated into a broader ADHD management plan, which may include behavioral therapy, medication, and lifestyle adjustments. It can be a tool to help children find moments of calm and focus in their daily lives.

Conclusion: Exploring Complementary Options

Aromatherapy offers a natural and soothing way to support children with ADHD. While it may not be a cure, it can be a valuable complementary approach to help manage symptoms and create a more relaxed and focused environment. As with any complementary therapy, it's essential to use essential oils safely and in conjunction with evidence-based treatments to provide the best possible support for children with ADHD.

Olfactory Memory and Emotional Well-Being: The Power of Scent in Nurturing Our Minds

Introduction:

The sense of smell, often overlooked in favor of sight and hearing, plays a profound role in our lives, influencing our emotions, memories, and overall well-being. Olfactory memory, the ability to recall memories and emotions triggered by scents, is a fascinating aspect of human psychology. In this comprehensive article, we will explore the connection between olfactory memory and emotional well-being, how scents impact our moods, and practical ways to harness the power of aroma for a healthier mind.

The Olfactory System: A Gateway to Memory and Emotion

The olfactory system, responsible for our sense of smell, is intricately linked to our brain's limbic system, which governs emotions, memories, and behavior. When we inhale a scent, the olfactory bulb, located at the base of the brain, processes the aroma and sends signals to various parts of the limbic system, including the amygdala and hippocampus. This process creates a powerful connection between scent, memory, and emotion.

Scent-Emotion Associations: Why Smells Trigger Feelings

Our brains form scent-emotion associations throughout our lives. For example, the aroma of freshly baked cookies may evoke feelings of warmth, comfort, and nostalgia because it's linked to positive childhood memories. In contrast, a scent associated with a traumatic event can trigger anxiety or distress. These associations are deeply rooted and can impact our emotional responses to scents in the present.

The Science of Aromatherapy: Impact on Mood and Well-Being

Aromatherapy, the practice of using essential oils and aromatic compounds to improve mental and physical health, harnesses the power of olfactory memory and scent-emotion associations. Various essential oils have been studied for their effects on mood and emotional well-being:

1. Lavender: Lavender oil is renowned for its calming properties and its ability to reduce stress and anxiety.

2. Citrus Oils (e.g., Orange, Lemon, Bergamot): Citrus scents are known for their uplifting and mood-enhancing effects.

3. Peppermint: Peppermint oil can boost alertness and focus, making it useful for productivity and concentration.

4. Rose: Rose oil is associated with feelings of love and positivity, promoting emotional balance.

5. Frankincense: Frankincense oil may aid in relaxation and deepening meditation practices.

Practical Ways to Harness Olfactory Memory for Well-Being:

1. Create Scented Rituals: Incorporate scents into daily routines, such as using lavender oil in your bedtime routine or citrus oils for morning invigoration.

2. Personal Fragrance: Choose perfumes or colognes with scents that evoke positive emotions for you. These can act as mood boosters throughout the day.

3. Aromatherapy Diffusers: Use diffusers to disperse essential oils in your living space, creating a calming or invigorating atmosphere as needed.

4. Scented Baths: Add a few drops of your favorite essential oil to your bath to relax and unwind.

5. Journaling: Keep a scent journal to record how different scents make you feel and any associated memories.

Conclusion: Nurturing Emotional Well-Being Through Scent

Understanding the profound connection between olfactory memory and emotional well-being allows us to use scent intentionally to enhance our moods and overall mental health. Whether through aromatherapy, personal fragrances, or simple daily rituals, the power of scent can be harnessed to reduce stress, boost positivity, and create a deeper connection with our emotions and memories. Embrace the world of olfactory memory, and let the aromatic treasures of life nurture your emotional well-being.

The Healing Properties of Blue Tansy Essential Oil

Introduction:

Blue Tansy essential oil, derived from the Moroccan Tansy plant (Tanacetum annuum), is gaining recognition for its remarkable healing properties and vibrant blue hue. This captivating oil, rich in a compound called chamazulene, offers a wide range of therapeutic benefits for both physical and emotional well-being. In this comprehensive article, we will explore the origins, chemical composition, and various uses of Blue Tansy essential oil, shedding light on its potential to promote healing and vitality.

A Glimpse into Blue Tansy: Origin and Extraction

Blue Tansy, also known as Moroccan Tansy or Tanacetum annuum, is a Mediterranean plant with yellow flowers. The essential oil is extracted from the aerial parts of the plant through a steam distillation process. What sets Blue Tansy apart is its unique blue color, which results from the presence of chamazulene, a potent anti-inflammatory compound.

Chemical Composition: The Magic of Chamazulene

The standout component in Blue Tansy essential oil is chamazulene, a chemical compound that forms during the distillation process from another compound called matricine. Chamazulene is renowned for its deep blue color and powerful anti-inflammatory and antioxidant properties. This compound is a key player in many of the healing benefits associated with Blue Tansy oil.

Healing Properties of Blue Tansy Essential Oil:

1. Anti-Inflammatory: Chamazulene's anti-inflammatory properties make Blue Tansy oil effective in reducing redness, swelling, and skin irritation. It can be used topically to soothe the skin conditions like eczema and dermatitis.

2. Antioxidant: Blue Tansy's high antioxidant content helps combat free radicals, protecting cells from oxidative damage and supporting overall health.

3. Pain Relief: The anti-inflammatory nature of Blue Tansy oil makes it a natural pain reliever. It can be diluted and applied topically to alleviate sore muscles and joints.

4. Respiratory Support: Inhaling the vapor of Blue Tansy oil can help relieve congestion and promote clear breathing during respiratory illnesses.

5. Emotional Balance: The soothing aroma of Blue Tansy oil can have a calming and grounding effect, making it useful for reducing stress and anxiety.

6. Skin Care: Blue Tansy oil is often used in skincare products due to its ability to promote a clear and radiant complexion. It can help balance oily or acne-prone skin.

Safe Usage and Dilution:

Blue Tansy oil is potent and should be used with care:

- Dilution: Always dilute Blue Tansy oil with a carrier oil (such as jojoba or coconut oil) before applying it to the skin. A common dilution ratio is 1-2 drops of Blue Tansy oil per ounce of carrier oil.

- Patch Test: Perform a patch test to check for skin sensitivities or allergies before applying it to larger areas of the skin.

- Aromatherapy: Diffusing Blue Tansy oil in an essential oil diffuser can help create a calming atmosphere. Use only a few drops.

- Consultation: If you have specific health concerns or are pregnant or nursing, consult with a healthcare professional before using Blue Tansy oil.

Conclusion: Embracing the Healing Power of Blue Tansy

Blue Tansy essential oil, with its vibrant color and remarkable healing properties, is a versatile addition to the world of natural remedies. Whether used for skincare, pain relief, emotional balance, or respiratory support, Blue Tansy's chamazulene-rich composition offers a wide range of therapeutic benefits. By understanding its safe usage and harnessing its healing potential, individuals can explore the captivating world of Blue Tansy essential oil to enhance their overall health and well-being.

Essential Oils for Dental Care: Fresh Breath and Healthy Gums

Introduction:

Maintaining good oral health is not only essential for a beautiful smile but also for overall well-being. Essential oils, with their natural antibacterial, anti-inflammatory, and aromatic properties, can be valuable allies in dental care. In this comprehensive article, we will delve into the world of essential oils for dental care, exploring their benefits, safe usage, and practical ways to promote fresh breath and healthy gums.

The Role of Essential Oils in Dental Care

Essential oils have been used for centuries in traditional medicine and oral hygiene practices. Their natural compounds make them effective for addressing various dental concerns:

1. Antibacterial: Many essential oils exhibit powerful antibacterial properties, which can help combat harmful bacteria in the mouth responsible for plaque, cavities, and gum disease.

2. Anti-Inflammatory: Some essential oils possess anti-inflammatory properties that can reduce gum inflammation and alleviate discomfort.

3. Aromatic: The pleasant scents of essential oils can combat bad breath, leaving your mouth feeling fresh and clean.

4. Antioxidant: Antioxidant-rich essential oils can help protect oral tissues from oxidative damage.

Top Essential Oils for Dental Care:

1. Peppermint (Mentha piperita): Peppermint oil is known for its fresh and invigorating aroma. It has antibacterial properties that combat odor-causing bacteria and promote fresh breath.

2. Tea Tree (Melaleuca alternifolia): Tea Tree oil is a potent antibacterial and antifungal agent. It can help reduce inflammation and combat gum disease.

3. Clove (Syzygium aromaticum): Clove oil is a natural analgesic and antiseptic. It can provide relief from toothaches and promote oral health.

4. Cinnamon (Cinnamomum verum): Cinnamon oil has antibacterial properties and a delightful, warm aroma. It can help combat bacteria and freshen breath.

5. Lemon (Citrus limon): Lemon oil has a refreshing citrus scent and is known for its antimicrobial properties. It can be used to combat bad breath.

Safe Usage of Essential Oils for Dental Care:

1. Dilution: Essential oils are highly concentrated and should be diluted before use. Mix a few drops with a carrier oil like coconut oil or water.

2. Oil Pulling: Oil pulling involves swishing diluted essential oils in your mouth for a few minutes. Spit it out afterward. This can help remove bacteria and debris.

3. Toothpaste or Mouthwash: Add a few drops of essential oil to your toothpaste or mouthwash for added benefits.

4. Oral Rinse: Create a homemade oral rinse by mixing water, a few drops of essential oil, and a pinch of salt. Rinse your mouth with it after brushing.

5. Diffusion: Use an essential oil diffuser with dental-friendly oils to freshen the air in your home.

Conclusion: Elevating Your Dental Care Routine

Essential oils offer a natural and effective way to enhance your dental care routine. Whether you're looking to combat bad breath, reduce gum inflammation, or promote overall oral health, essential oils can be valuable additions to your toolkit. By understanding their benefits and safe usage, you can harness the power of nature to achieve fresh breath and maintain healthy gums, contributing to a radiant smile and improved well-being.

The Spiritual Significance of Oud Essential Oil

Introduction:

Oud, also known as agarwood or aloeswood, is a resinous heartwood that holds great spiritual and cultural significance across various cultures and religions. Extracted from the Aquilaria tree, Oud essential oil is renowned for its rich, woody aroma and its association with spirituality, meditation, and well-being. In this comprehensive article, we will delve into the spiritual significance of Oud essential oil, its historical and cultural roots, and its modern applications for enhancing spiritual experiences.

The Mystique of Oud: Origins and Production

Oud is not an ordinary essential oil; it is a rare and precious substance that forms in the heartwood of the Aquilaria tree when it becomes infected with a specific type of mold. This infection triggers a natural defense mechanism within the tree, leading to the formation of resin-rich agarwood. The resin is then steam-distilled to create Oud essential oil.

Historical and Cultural Significance:

1. Ancient Roots: Oud's history dates back thousands of years, with references in ancient texts, such as the Vedas and the Bible. It has been used in spiritual rituals, ceremonies, and perfumery.

2. Spiritual Practices: Oud has been used in various spiritual and religious practices. In Buddhism, it is considered one of the most sacred scents and is often used as an offering to the Buddha. In Islam, it is mentioned in the Hadith and is used as a perfume during prayer.

3. Meditation and Mindfulness: Oud's deep, grounding scent is believed to aid meditation and mindfulness practices by promoting a sense of tranquility, focus, and spiritual connection.

Modern Applications for Spiritual Well-Being:

1. Aromatherapy: Oud essential oil is used in aromatherapy to create an atmosphere of serenity and inner peace. It is often diffused or used in personal inhalers during meditation and relaxation exercises.

2. Perfumery: Oud's unique and complex fragrance is highly sought after in the perfume industry. Wearing Oud-based perfumes or attar (traditional Middle Eastern perfume) can evoke a sense of spirituality and connection to nature.

3. Spiritual Retreats: Oud is sometimes incorporated into spiritual retreats and wellness practices to enhance the experience of participants. Its aroma is believed to facilitate introspection and spiritual growth.

4. Cleansing and Purification: Oud smoke has been used for centuries in purification rituals. Burning Oud chips or incense sticks can cleanse spaces of negative energy and promote positive vibrations.

Safe and Ethical Usage:

Due to its rarity and high demand, Oud can be expensive and is sometimes subject to unethical practices. It's important to source Oud from reputable suppliers who adhere to sustainable and ethical harvesting methods.

Conclusion: A Journey of Spirituality and Serenity

Oud essential oil, with its deep-rooted spiritual significance and captivating aroma, continues to be cherished in contemporary society. Whether used in meditation, perfumery, or spiritual rituals, Oud has the power to transport individuals to a state of inner peace and connection to the divine. By understanding its historical and cultural context and practicing ethical sourcing, we can embark on a fragrant journey of spirituality and serenity with Oud as our guide.

The Role of Essential Oils in Hospice Care

Introduction:

Hospice care focuses on providing comfort and support to individuals facing terminal illnesses, enhancing their quality of life during their final journey. Essential oils, with their holistic and non-invasive nature, have found a meaningful place in hospice care. In this comprehensive article, we will explore the role of essential oils in hospice care, their benefits for patients and their families, and the sensitive approach required for their use in end-of-life situations.

Comfort and Emotional Support:

1. Pain Management: Some essential oils, such as lavender and peppermint, have analgesic properties that can help alleviate pain and discomfort, offering relief to patients who may be experiencing physical distress.

2. Anxiety and Stress Reduction: Essential oils like chamomile and frankincense can promote relaxation and reduce anxiety, helping patients cope with the emotional challenges of end-of-life care.

3. Improved Sleep: Lavender and cedarwood essential oils are known for their calming effects, which can aid in improving the sleep quality of both patients and their caregivers.

4. Emotional Support: Aromatherapy with essential oils can provide emotional support by creating a soothing and nurturing environment, fostering a sense of comfort and peace.

Symptom Management:

1. Nausea and Vomiting: Ginger and peppermint essential oils have antiemetic properties that can help manage nausea and vomiting, common symptoms in hospice patients.

2. Respiratory Support: Eucalyptus and tea tree oils can be diffused or applied topically to relieve congestion and facilitate easier breathing, providing comfort to patients with respiratory issues.

Practical Applications:

1. Aromatherapy Diffusion: Essential oil diffusers are often used in hospice settings to disperse soothing scents throughout patient rooms, common areas, and even in relaxation spaces.

2. Massage and Topical Applications: Diluted essential oils can be gently massaged onto a patient's skin, providing both physical and emotional comfort. This tactile approach can enhance the sense of human connection.

3. Personal Inhalers: Patients and family members can use personal inhalers infused with comforting essential oils to provide quick access to emotional support during moments of distress.

Special Considerations and Ethical Practices:

1. Patient Preferences: It's essential to consider individual patient preferences and sensitivities when using essential oils. Some patients may have allergies or aversions to certain scents.

2. Open Communication: Hospice care providers should maintain open and honest communication with patients and their families regarding the use of essential oils and respect their choices.

3. Ethical Sourcing: Ensure that the essential oils used in hospice care are ethically sourced and of high quality. Organic and therapeutic-grade oils are often preferred.

Conclusion: Enhancing End-of-Life Care with Compassion

Essential oils have become valuable tools in the realm of hospice care, offering a compassionate and holistic approach to end-of-life support. By addressing both physical symptoms and emotional needs, these aromatic allies provide comfort and solace to patients and their families during a profoundly challenging time. The use of essential oils in hospice care exemplifies the importance of holistic care that acknowledges the mind, body, and spirit, allowing individuals to find peace and comfort in their final moments.

Crafting Essential Oil Room Sprays for Mood Enhancement

Introduction:

The power of scent to influence our emotions and mood is undeniable. Essential oils, with their diverse and captivating fragrances, offer an exciting avenue for mood enhancement. Crafting your own essential oil room sprays allows you to personalize your surroundings and uplift your spirits. In this detailed guide, we will explore the art of creating essential oil room sprays that can transform your environment and create a positive atmosphere.

Getting Started: Essential Oils and Their Effects

Before you start mixing, it's essential to understand the emotional effects of different essential oils. Here are some popular choices and their mood-enhancing properties:

1. Lavender: Calming and soothing, ideal for relaxation and stress reduction.

2. Citrus Oils (Lemon, Orange, Grapefruit): Energizing and mood-lifting, perfect for a cheerful ambiance.

3. Peppermint: Invigorating and refreshing, great for boosting focus and alertness.

4. Ylang-Ylang: Romantic and sensual, suitable for creating a romantic atmosphere.

5. Eucalyptus: Uplifting and clearing, excellent for promoting a sense of clarity.

Creating Your Essential Oil Room Spray:

Ingredients:

- 2 oz (60 ml) spray bottle
- Distilled water or witch hazel as a base
- Essential oils of your choice (usually 15-20 drops in total)
- Optional: A small amount of alcohol (vodka or rubbing alcohol) to help disperse the oils evenly in the water

Steps:

1. Choose Your Oils: Decide which essential oils you want to use based on the mood you want to create. You can use a single oil or create a blend.

2. Calculate Drops: Determine the total number of drops needed. A general guideline is 15-20 drops of essential oil for a 2 oz spray bottle. You can adjust the ratio to your preference.

3. Mixing: Add the essential oil drops to your empty spray bottle. If you're using alcohol, add it first to help disperse the oils evenly.

4. Adding Base: Fill the spray bottle almost to the top with distilled water or witch hazel. Leave some space at the top for easy mixing.

5. Shake Well: Secure the spray cap and shake the bottle vigorously to mix the essential oils with the base.

6. Testing: Spray a small amount into the air to test the aroma. If it's too strong, you can dilute it further with more water.

Customizing Your Room Spray:

The beauty of crafting your own room sprays is the ability to customize them according to your preferences. You can experiment with different essential oil combinations until you find the perfect blend for your desired mood or occasion.

Storage and Usage:

- Store your room spray in a cool, dark place to preserve the integrity of the essential oils.

- Shake well before each use to ensure the oils are evenly distributed.

- Use your room spray to freshen up any space: bedrooms, living rooms, bathrooms, and even your car.

- Spritz a little on linens or pillows for a soothing bedtime routine.

Conclusion: Aroma, Mood, and Personal Well-Being

Crafting essential oil room sprays is not only a creative endeavor but also a way to enhance your environment and influence your mood positively. Whether you seek relaxation, energy, or a touch of romance, the right blend of essential oils can transform any space into a sanctuary of well-being. By experimenting with different scents and creating your unique combinations, you can enjoy the benefits of aromatherapy and elevate your daily life with the power of scent.

Patchouli Essential Oil: From Hippies to Holistic Healing

Introduction:

Patchouli essential oil, with its earthy, exotic aroma, has a storied history that spans continents and cultures. While often associated with the counterculture movements of the 1960s, patchouli has a much deeper heritage and a wide range of holistic healing properties. In this comprehensive article, we will explore the fascinating journey of patchouli essential oil from its origins to its contemporary uses in holistic wellness.

Aromatic Origins:

Patchouli (Pogostemon cablin) is a tropical perennial plant native to Southeast Asia, particularly Indonesia and the Philippines. The essential oil is extracted from the leaves of the patchouli plant through steam distillation. It is renowned for its distinctive and complex scent, described as earthy, sweet, and musky.

Historical Significance:

1. Ancient India: Patchouli has deep roots in Ayurvedic medicine, where it was used for its calming and grounding properties. It was also used as a moth repellent for textiles.

2. Silk Road Trade: Along the ancient Silk Road, patchouli leaves were packed with valuable textiles to protect them from insects and impart a pleasant aroma.

The Hippie Movement:

Patchouli became an iconic scent of the 1960s counterculture, associated with peace, love, and individuality. Hippies wore patchouli-scented clothing and used the oil as a fragrance, which led to its nickname as the "hippie perfume."

Holistic Healing Properties:

1. Emotional Balance: Patchouli is known for its grounding and emotionally stabilizing effects. It can help reduce anxiety, stress, and feelings of overwhelm.

2. Skin Health: Patchouli essential oil has antiseptic and anti-inflammatory properties, making it useful for treating minor skin irritations, acne, and wounds.

3. Aphrodisiac: In aromatherapy, patchouli is considered an aphrodisiac that can enhance sensuality and intimacy.

4. Insect Repellent: Just as it was used in ancient times, patchouli remains an effective natural insect repellent.

Modern Applications:

1. Aromatherapy: Patchouli is used in aromatherapy to promote relaxation, emotional balance, and stress relief. It can be diffused or diluted and applied topically.

2. Skincare: Many natural skincare products incorporate patchouli for its skin-healing properties. It can help with acne, eczema, and general skin health.

3. Perfumery: Patchouli's unique scent is a valuable component in perfumery. It is often used as a base note to anchor fragrances.

Ethical Considerations:

Sustainable and ethical sourcing of patchouli essential oil is crucial. Overharvesting has led to ecological concerns, and responsible cultivation practices are essential for its preservation.

Conclusion: A Fragrant Tapestry of History and Healing

Patchouli essential oil is a remarkable example of a plant with a diverse and culturally rich history. From its origins in Ayurvedic medicine to its iconic role in the hippie movement, patchouli has left an indelible mark on both fragrance and holistic wellness. Today, it continues to be a beloved essential oil with a wide range of applications in aromatherapy, skincare, and perfumery. The journey of patchouli is a testament to the enduring power of scent and its ability to connect us to our past while enriching our present.

Aromatherapy for Senior Citizens: Enhancing Later Years

Introduction:

Aromatherapy, the practice of using essential oils for therapeutic purposes, has gained recognition for its potential to enhance the well-being of individuals in various life stages. For senior citizens, aromatherapy offers a gentle and holistic approach to addressing common challenges associated with aging, promoting relaxation, and supporting overall health. In this comprehensive article, we will explore the benefits of aromatherapy for senior citizens and provide practical tips for its safe and effective use.

Understanding the Unique Needs of Senior Citizens:

As individuals age, they encounter a range of physical, emotional, and cognitive changes. Aromatherapy can be tailored to address the specific needs and challenges faced by senior citizens:

1. Pain Management: Many seniors experience chronic pain conditions. Certain essential oils, such as lavender and eucalyptus, have analgesic properties that can offer relief.

2. Cognitive Health: Cognitive decline is a concern for some seniors. Rosemary and peppermint essential oils are known for their potential to improve focus and memory.

3. Emotional Well-Being: Loneliness, depression, and anxiety can affect seniors' mental health. Aromatherapy can provide emotional support and uplift spirits.

4. Sleep Disturbances: Sleep disorders are common among older adults. Lavender and chamomile essential oils can promote relaxation and improve sleep quality.

5. Respiratory Health: Seniors may face respiratory challenges. Eucalyptus and tea tree oils can assist in clearing congestion and supporting respiratory well-being.

Benefits of Aromatherapy for Senior Citizens:

1. Stress Reduction: Aromatherapy can help seniors manage stress and anxiety, promoting a sense of calm and relaxation.

2. Improved Sleep: Certain essential oils can create a soothing bedtime routine, leading to better sleep quality and overall rest.

3. Enhanced Mood: Aromatherapy can uplift spirits and combat feelings of loneliness or depression, enhancing emotional well-being.

4. Pain Relief: Essential oils with analgesic properties can offer relief from chronic pain conditions, promoting comfort.

5. Improved Cognitive Function: Aromatherapy can potentially support cognitive function, aiding memory and focus.

Practical Tips for Using Aromatherapy with Seniors:

1. Dilution: Essential oils should be properly diluted in a carrier oil before use to avoid skin irritation.

2. Diffusion: Aromatherapy diffusers can create a gentle and consistent aroma in living spaces.

3. Topical Application: For localized pain relief or targeted benefits, essential oils can be diluted and applied topically. Always perform a patch test first.

4. Bedtime Routine: Incorporate aromatherapy into a calming bedtime routine to improve sleep quality.

5. Open Communication: Consult with healthcare professionals when using aromatherapy, especially if seniors have underlying health conditions or are on medications.

Conclusion: A Gentle Path to Well-Being

Aromatherapy offers a gentle and holistic approach to enhancing the well-being of senior citizens. Its potential benefits for stress reduction, sleep improvement, pain relief, and emotional support make it a valuable addition to the care and quality of life of older adults. By understanding the unique needs of senior citizens and using aromatherapy safely and effectively, caregivers and seniors themselves can embark on a fragrant journey towards enhanced well-being in later years.

The Benefits of Cypress Oil for Circulation and Respiration

Introduction:

Cypress oil, derived from the branches and needles of the cypress tree (Cupressus sempervirens), is a versatile essential oil known for its numerous therapeutic properties. Among its many uses, cypress oil stands out as a natural remedy for improving circulation and supporting respiratory health. In this detailed article, we will explore the benefits and applications of cypress oil in promoting optimal circulation and respiratory well-being.

Understanding Cypress Oil:

Cypress oil has a fresh, woody aroma with subtle hints of pine and lemon. It has been used for centuries in traditional medicine and aromatherapy for its healing properties. Here, we focus on two key areas where cypress oil shines:

1. Circulation Enhancement:

Benefits:

1. Improved Blood Flow: Cypress oil is a vasodilator, meaning it widens blood vessels, which can lead to improved blood circulation. This can

be particularly beneficial for individuals with poor circulation or those experiencing cold extremities.

2. Reduction of Varicose Veins: Cypress oil's vasoconstrictive properties help reduce the appearance of varicose veins and spider veins by tightening blood vessels.

3. Hemorrhoid Relief: Cypress oil's vasoconstrictor abilities can also alleviate the discomfort associated with hemorrhoids.

2. Respiratory Support:

Benefits:

1. Decongestant: Cypress oil acts as a natural decongestant, making it effective for clearing nasal and bronchial congestion.

2. Cough Relief: It can help alleviate coughs by loosening mucus and promoting easier breathing.

3. Antispasmodic: Cypress oil's antispasmodic properties can help relax respiratory muscles, reducing symptoms of conditions like asthma.

How to Use Cypress Oil for Circulation and Respiration:

1. Topical Application: For circulation, dilute a few drops of cypress oil in a carrier oil (such as coconut or jojoba) and massage it onto the skin. For respiratory support, apply diluted oil to the chest or add a few drops to a bowl of hot water for steam inhalation.

2. Aromatherapy: Diffuse cypress oil in your home or workplace to benefit from its aromatic properties. The diffused aroma can help reduce stress and anxiety while supporting respiratory health.

3. Bath Soak: Add a few drops of cypress oil to your bathwater for a relaxing and circulation-boosting soak.

4. Compress: Soak a cloth in warm water with a few drops of cypress oil and apply it as a compress to areas with poor circulation or respiratory discomfort.

Safety Considerations:

- Cypress oil is generally safe for topical use when properly diluted, but a patch test is recommended to check for skin sensitivity.

- Pregnant or breastfeeding women and individuals with certain medical conditions should consult with a healthcare professional before using cypress oil.

Conclusion: Cypress Oil, Nature's Support for Circulation and Breathing

Cypress oil's versatility makes it a valuable addition to your holistic health toolkit. Whether you seek to enhance circulation, reduce the appearance of varicose veins, or support respiratory wellness, cypress oil offers a natural and fragrant solution. By harnessing the power of this remarkable essential oil, you can embark on a journey towards improved circulation and easier, deeper breaths, leading to a greater sense of well-being and vitality.

Essential Oils for Allergy Relief: Tackling Seasonal Sniffles

Introduction:

Seasonal allergies, characterized by sneezing, runny noses, itchy eyes, and congestion, can significantly impact one's quality of life. While over-the-counter medications are commonly used to manage allergy symptoms, many individuals seek natural alternatives like essential oils to alleviate their discomfort. In this comprehensive article, we will explore how essential oils can offer effective relief from seasonal allergies and improve overall well-being.

Understanding Seasonal Allergies:

Seasonal allergies, also known as hay fever or allergic rhinitis, occur when the immune system overreacts to pollen from trees, grasses, weeds, or mold spores. Common symptoms include:

- Sneezing
- Runny or stuffy nose
- Itchy or watery eyes
- Coughing
- Fatigue

The Role of Essential Oils in Allergy Relief:

Essential oils are concentrated extracts from plants that contain compounds known for their anti-inflammatory, antihistamine, and immune-modulating properties. When used appropriately, they can help alleviate the symptoms of seasonal allergies and provide relief without the side effects associated with some medications.

Top Essential Oils for Allergy Relief:

1. Lavender Oil: Lavender has anti-inflammatory properties and can help reduce inflammation in the nasal passages and calm the body's response to allergens.

2. Peppermint Oil: Peppermint is a natural decongestant and can open up airways, making breathing easier for allergy sufferers.

3. Eucalyptus Oil: Eucalyptus has antimicrobial and anti-inflammatory properties and can relieve nasal congestion.

4. Tea Tree Oil: Tea tree oil has anti-inflammatory and antiseptic properties, which can help reduce symptoms and prevent secondary infections.

5. Chamomile Oil: Chamomile has anti-inflammatory and antihistamine properties and can soothe irritated skin and mucous membranes.

How to Use Essential Oils for Allergy Relief:

1. Diffusion: Add a few drops of your chosen essential oil to a diffuser and let it run in your living space. This method can help reduce airborne allergens and create a more pleasant environment.

2. Topical Application: Dilute essential oils with a carrier oil (such as coconut oil) and apply to the chest, temples, or under the nose. Ensure proper dilution to avoid skin irritation.

3. Steam Inhalation: Add a few drops of essential oil to a bowl of hot water, lean over it with a towel draped over your head, and inhale the steam. This can help clear nasal passages and reduce congestion.

4. Aromatic Bath: Adding essential oils to a warm bath can provide relief by promoting relaxation and reducing inflammation.

Safety Considerations:

- Always dilute essential oils before applying them to the skin, especially for individuals with sensitive skin.

- Perform a patch test to check for allergies or skin sensitivities.

- Consult with a healthcare professional, especially if you have underlying health conditions or are taking medications.

Conclusion: Natural Allergy Relief with Essential Oils

Seasonal allergies can be a source of discomfort and annoyance, but essential oils offer a natural and effective way to manage symptoms and improve your overall well-being. By harnessing the power of lavender, peppermint, eucalyptus, tea tree, chamomile, and other essential oils, you can find relief from seasonal sniffles and enjoy the benefits of a more comfortable and symptom-free life during allergy season. Always use essential oils with care and seek guidance from a healthcare professional when needed for safe and effective allergy management.

Creating Essential Oil Roll-On Blends for On-the-Go Use

Introduction:

Essential oils have gained immense popularity for their therapeutic properties and versatility. One convenient and portable way to enjoy the benefits of essential oils is by creating roll-on blends. These small, travel-friendly bottles contain diluted essential oils that can be easily applied to the skin. In this detailed article, we'll explore the art of making essential oil roll-on blends for on-the-go use, providing you with tips, recipes, and safety guidelines to craft your personalized aromatic companions.

Why Choose Roll-On Blends?

Roll-on blends offer several advantages:

1. Ease of Application: Roll-ons are mess-free and easy to apply directly to the skin, making them ideal for busy lifestyles.

2. Portability: They fit comfortably in pockets, purses, or backpacks, allowing you to carry your favorite essential oils wherever you go.

3. Customization: You have the freedom to create personalized blends tailored to your specific needs and preferences.

Materials Needed:

1. Essential Oils: Choose high-quality essential oils known for their therapeutic properties. Popular choices include lavender, peppermint, eucalyptus, tea tree, and more.

2. Carrier Oil: A carrier oil, such as fractionated coconut oil, jojoba oil, or sweet almond oil, is used to dilute essential oils and make them safe for skin application.

3. Roll-On Bottles: Purchase roll-on bottles with rollerball applicators for easy application. These can be found in various sizes, from 5ml to 10ml, to suit your needs.

4. Labels: Labeling your roll-on blends is essential to keep track of the oils used and their intended purposes.

Steps to Create Essential Oil Roll-On Blends:

1. Choose Your Blend: Decide on the purpose of your blend, whether it's for relaxation, energy, focus, or skin care. Each blend will require different essential oils.

2. Select Essential Oils: Research the therapeutic properties of essential oils and select those that align with your blend's purpose. For example, lavender and chamomile are excellent for relaxation.

3. Dilution: Dilute essential oils in a carrier oil. A common dilution ratio is 2-3% essential oil to carrier oil for adults. For a 10ml roll-on bottle, this equates to about 6-9 drops of essential oil.

4. Blending: Combine your chosen essential oils and carrier oil in a separate container. Start with a small quantity, and adjust the scent by adding more essential oils if needed.

5. Filling the Bottle: Use a dropper or a small funnel to transfer your blend into the roll-on bottle. Leave a small gap at the top to avoid spills when inserting the rollerball.

6. Insert the Rollerball: Carefully insert the rollerball into the bottle, ensuring it's securely in place.

7. Labeling: Label your roll-on bottle with the blend's name and purpose. Include the date of creation for reference.

8. Storage: Store your roll-on blends in a cool, dark place to preserve their potency.

Safety Guidelines:

- Always dilute essential oils before applying them to the skin to prevent irritation or sensitization.

- Perform a patch test to check for allergic reactions or skin sensitivity before widespread use.

- Consult with a healthcare professional, especially if you are pregnant, nursing, or have underlying health conditions.

Roll-On Blend Recipes:

1. Calming Blend:

   - 4 drops lavender

   - 3 drops chamomile

   - 10ml carrier oil

2. Energizing Blend:

   - 4 drops peppermint

   - 3 drops lemon

   - 10ml carrier oil

3. Focus Blend:

   - 4 drops rosemary

   - 3 drops frankincense

- 10ml carrier oil

4. Skin Soothing Blend:
   - 4 drops tea tree
   - 3 drops lavender
   - 10ml carrier oil

Conclusion: Your Personal Aromatic Companions

Creating essential oil roll-on blends is a delightful and practical way to incorporate aromatherapy into your daily routine. Whether you seek relaxation, energy, focus, or skin care, these portable blends are ready to provide the aromatic support you need, wherever you go. By following safety guidelines and experimenting with different essential oil combinations, you can craft personalized roll-on blends that become your trusted companions for on-the-go well-being.

The Aromas of Ancient Rome: Oils in Baths and Perfumes

Introduction:

The use of essential oils and aromatic substances is a practice that spans millennia and transcends cultures. In ancient Rome, the art of perfumery and bathing reached remarkable sophistication, and essential oils played a pivotal role in daily life. In this detailed article, we delve into the aromatic world of ancient Rome, exploring how oils were utilized in baths, perfumes, and everyday rituals, shedding light on a fragrance-rich era that continues to influence modern perfumery.

The Roman Bathing Culture:

Bathing was a sacred ritual for the ancient Romans, central to their daily lives and social interactions. Public bathhouses, called "thermae," were opulent structures where people gathered not only for hygiene but also for leisure, relaxation, and socializing. Essential oils were integral to this experience in several ways:

1. Aromatic Baths:

Roman baths were scented havens, with fragrant oils diffused in the air and infused in the bathwater. Oils like rose, lavender, and myrtle were popular choices. These aromatic baths were believed to cleanse the body and rejuvenate the spirit, providing a multisensory experience.

2. Perfumed Oils:

Roman women and men alike indulged in fragrant oils and unguents (ointments) to scent their bodies. Essential oils were blended with base oils, such as olive or almond oil, to create personalized perfumes. These scents were applied not only for personal enjoyment but also as a status symbol.

3. Rituals of Purification:

The Romans believed that essential oils possessed purifying properties. Before entering a bath, individuals would often anoint themselves with fragrant oils to prepare for the cleansing ritual. These oils were thought to protect against evil spirits and promote well-being.

Roman Perfumery:

Perfumery was an esteemed craft in ancient Rome, and perfumers, known as "unguentarii," were highly regarded artisans. They created a wide array of scented products, including solid perfumes, oils, and balms. Here are some key aspects of Roman perfumery:

1. Natural Ingredients:

Roman perfumers sourced their ingredients from various regions of the empire. They used a wide range of aromatic materials, including flowers like roses and lilies, resins like frankincense and myrrh, and spices like cinnamon and cardamom.

2. Extraction Methods:

The Romans employed various methods to extract aromatic compounds from plants, including steam distillation and maceration. These techniques allowed them to create a diverse array of scents.

3. Scented Fashion:

Perfumes were applied not only to the skin but also to clothing and even hairpieces. The Romans infused their clothing with fragrances, and it was common to find perfumed sachets in their wardrobes.

4. Symbolism and Ritual:

Scented oils and perfumes held symbolic meaning in Roman society. They were given as gifts, used in religious ceremonies, and even applied to statues and offerings to the gods.

Legacy and Influence:

The legacy of Roman perfumery and bathing culture continues to influence modern fragrance practices. The use of essential oils in perfumery, skincare, and aromatherapy can be traced back to the aromatic traditions of ancient Rome. Today, we still appreciate the sensory delights of scented baths and perfumes, and we owe a debt to the Romans for laying the fragrant foundation.

Conclusion: A Fragrant Heritage

The Romans' deep appreciation for the art of perfumery and the therapeutic benefits of essential oils left an indelible mark on history. Their use of oils in baths and perfumes not only elevated their daily lives but also contributed to the development of modern fragrance practices. As we continue to explore the world of aromatics and their role in well-being, we can draw inspiration from the aromatic heritage of ancient Rome, where the power of fragrance was celebrated in its most exquisite form.

Thyme Essential Oil: A Potent Antibacterial and Antiviral Agent

Introduction:

Thyme essential oil, derived from the aromatic herb Thymus vulgaris, has a long history of culinary and medicinal use. Beyond its delightful flavor, thyme oil possesses powerful antibacterial and antiviral properties that have made it a valuable tool in traditional medicine and modern aromatherapy. In this comprehensive article, we will explore the fascinating world of thyme essential oil, delving into its history, composition, health benefits, and practical applications.

A Brief History of Thyme:

Thyme is an herb native to the Mediterranean region and has been utilized for thousands of years in various cultures. The ancient Egyptians used thyme in embalming practices, while the ancient Greeks employed it for its aromatic and medicinal qualities. In medieval Europe, thyme was a staple in herb gardens and found its way into herbal remedies for ailments ranging from respiratory conditions to digestive issues.

The Composition of Thyme Essential Oil:

Thyme essential oil owes its remarkable properties to its complex chemical composition, which includes:

1. Thymol: Thymol is the primary bioactive compound in thyme oil, responsible for its strong antimicrobial properties.

2. Carvacrol: Carvacrol is another significant component known for its antibacterial and antifungal properties.

3. P-Cymene: This compound contributes to thyme oil's antimicrobial activity and is also found in other essential oils like cumin and oregano.

4. Linalool: Linalool provides thyme oil with a pleasant aroma and has soothing properties.

Health Benefits of Thyme Essential Oil:

1. Antibacterial Action: Thyme essential oil has been shown to inhibit the growth of various bacteria, making it a valuable tool in natural cleaning products and for addressing bacterial infections.

2. Antiviral Properties: Thyme oil's antiviral activity makes it useful for combating viral infections like the common cold and flu.

3. Respiratory Relief: Thyme oil is often used to alleviate respiratory issues such as coughs, bronchitis, and congestion. It can be inhaled directly or used in steam inhalation.

4. Immune Support: Thyme oil's immune-boosting properties can help the body defend against infections and promote overall wellness.

5. Skin Health: Thyme oil may aid in treating skin conditions like acne due to its antimicrobial properties. It should be used with caution on the skin and properly diluted.

Practical Applications:

1. Aromatherapy: Diffusing thyme essential oil in your home can help purify the air and support respiratory health.

2. Massage: When diluted with a carrier oil, thyme oil can be used in a soothing massage to relieve muscle tension and support overall well-being.

3. Topical Application: Carefully diluted thyme oil can be applied topically to treat skin issues or as a natural antibacterial agent for minor cuts and wounds.

4. Steam Inhalation: Inhaling thyme oil vapor by adding a few drops to a bowl of hot water can help clear congested airways and relieve cold symptoms.

Safety Considerations:

Thyme essential oil is potent and should be used with care:

- Always dilute thyme oil with a suitable carrier oil before applying it to the skin.

- Perform a patch test to check for any skin sensitivity or allergies.

- Avoid using undiluted thyme oil on children, pregnant individuals, or those with sensitive skin.

- Consult with a healthcare professional before using thyme oil for medical purposes, especially if you have underlying health conditions or are taking medications.

Conclusion: Nature's Antibacterial Ally

Thyme essential oil is a testament to the power of nature in providing potent antibacterial and antiviral solutions. Its rich history and versatile applications make it a valuable addition to your holistic wellness toolkit. Whether diffused in your living space, used in massage blends, or applied topically for skin concerns, thyme essential oil offers a natural and aromatic approach to promoting health and vitality. Always remember to use it mindfully, with a deep appreciation for its potent properties and historical significance.

Essential Oils for Alzheimer's and Dementia Support: A Holistic Approach

Introduction:

Alzheimer's disease and other forms of dementia can profoundly affect individuals and their families. While there is no cure for these conditions, holistic approaches that incorporate essential oils have gained attention for their potential to improve the well-being and quality of life for those living with Alzheimer's and dementia. In this comprehensive article, we will explore the use of essential oils in Alzheimer's and dementia care, including their benefits, safety considerations, and practical applications.

Understanding Alzheimer's and Dementia:

Alzheimer's disease is a progressive brain disorder that affects memory, cognitive function, and behavior. Dementia is an umbrella term encompassing various cognitive impairments, with Alzheimer's being the most common form. Individuals with Alzheimer's and dementia often experience anxiety, depression, agitation, and sleep disturbances.

The Role of Essential Oils:

Essential oils are concentrated extracts from plants that contain aromatic compounds with potential therapeutic properties. When used mindfully, essential oils can offer emotional and psychological support for individuals with Alzheimer's and dementia. Here are some ways they can help:

1. Aromatherapy for Emotional Well-being:

Aromatherapy, the use of essential oils for therapeutic purposes, can help alleviate emotional distress often associated with dementia. Certain essential oils, such as lavender, chamomile, and rosemary, have calming and mood-lifting properties. Diffusing these oils in the living space or using them in a personal inhaler can promote a sense of peace and well-being.

2. Memory Enhancement:

While essential oils cannot reverse memory loss, some aromas may stimulate memory recall. Rosemary essential oil, for instance, has been linked to improved memory retention and cognitive function. Inhalation of rosemary oil can be integrated into daily routines or during memory-related activities.

3. Stress and Anxiety Reduction:

Lavender and bergamot essential oils are well-known for their anxiety-reducing effects. Diffusing these oils or using them in massage blends can help manage stress and anxiety in individuals with dementia.

4. Improved Sleep:

Sleep disturbances are common among individuals with Alzheimer's and dementia. Essential oils like lavender and cedarwood have sedative properties that can promote better sleep. A few drops on a pillow or in a diffuser before bedtime can support a more restful night's sleep.

5. Communication and Engagement:

Engaging in sensory activities with essential oils can foster communication and connection. Encouraging individuals to touch and explore scented objects or participate in aromatherapy sessions can enhance their quality of life.

Safety Considerations:

When using essential oils for Alzheimer's and dementia support, it's crucial to prioritize safety:

- Dilution: Essential oils should always be properly diluted in a carrier oil before applying to the skin, especially for massage.
- Patch Testing: Perform a patch test on a small area of skin to check for any adverse reactions or allergies.
- Consultation: Consult with a healthcare professional, such as a qualified aromatherapist or a physician, before using essential oils,

especially if the individual has underlying health conditions or is taking medications.

Practical Applications:

1. Aromatherapy Diffusion: Use an essential oil diffuser to disperse calming scents in the living space. Consider diffusing lavender, bergamot, or frankincense.

2. Massage: Gentle, aromatherapy massage with diluted essential oils can provide relaxation and tactile comfort.

3. Personal Inhalers: Create personal inhalers with calming oils for on-the-go emotional support.

4. Scented Objects: Fill sachets or small bags with fragrant herbs and place them in drawers or pillows.

5. Sensory Activities: Engage individuals with dementia in sensory activities, such as smelling various essential oils, as part of their daily routine.

Conclusion: Enhancing Quality of Life

While essential oils cannot cure Alzheimer's or dementia, they offer a holistic and complementary approach to support emotional well-being and alleviate distressing symptoms. Caregivers, healthcare professionals, and family members can work together to integrate aromatherapy safely into the care routines of individuals living with these conditions. By focusing on emotional comfort and engagement, essential oils can enhance the quality of life for both those with dementia and their caregivers.

Aromatherapy in the Workplace: Reducing Stress and Boosting Productivity

Introduction:

The modern workplace is often characterized by high demands, tight deadlines, and a fast-paced environment that can lead to stress and burnout. Aromatherapy, the use of essential oils for therapeutic purposes, has gained popularity as a natural and effective way to alleviate stress and enhance productivity in the workplace. In this comprehensive article, we will explore the benefits of aromatherapy in professional settings, practical applications, and strategies for creating a more pleasant and productive work environment.

Understanding Workplace Stress:

Work-related stress is a common issue affecting employees across various industries. It can manifest as physical symptoms, such as headaches and muscle tension, as well as emotional challenges like anxiety and fatigue. Prolonged stress not only impacts well-being but can also reduce productivity and job satisfaction.

The Benefits of Aromatherapy in the Workplace:

Aromatherapy offers a range of benefits that make it a valuable tool for addressing workplace stress:

1. Stress Reduction:

Certain essential oils, such as lavender, chamomile, and frankincense, have calming properties that can help reduce stress and anxiety levels among employees. Diffusing these oils in the workplace creates a soothing atmosphere.

2. Improved Focus and Concentration:

Peppermint, rosemary, and lemon essential oils are known for their invigorating and mentally clarifying effects. Inhaling these scents can enhance concentration and cognitive function, making employees more productive.

3. Enhanced Mood and Well-being:

Aromas like citrus and floral scents have mood-lifting properties that can create a more positive and pleasant work environment. Improved mood can lead to greater job satisfaction.

4. Increased Energy and Vitality:

Fatigue and lethargy can be common workplace issues. Essential oils like eucalyptus and ginger can provide a natural energy boost when diffused or applied topically.

5. Stress Management Tools:

Aromatherapy provides employees with practical stress management tools they can use independently, such as personal inhalers or roll-on blends, to address stress as needed.

Practical Applications in the Workplace:

1. Diffusers: Use essential oil diffusers in common areas or individual workspaces to disperse aromas throughout the day. Consider a variety of scents to cater to different preferences.

2. Desk Blends: Employees can create personal aromatherapy blends in rollerball bottles, allowing them to apply oils directly to their pulse points for quick stress relief.

3. Meeting Rooms: Infuse meeting rooms with invigorating scents like rosemary and lemon to promote alertness and creativity during brainstorming sessions.

4. Wellness Programs: Incorporate aromatherapy into workplace wellness programs by offering workshops or educational sessions on the benefits of essential oils and how to use them safely.

Creating a Supportive Aromatherapy Environment:

To effectively implement aromatherapy in the workplace, consider the following strategies:

- Employee Input: Gather feedback from employees about their preferred scents and any sensitivities or allergies to ensure a comfortable environment.

- Safety First: Educate employees about the safe use of essential oils, including proper dilution and potential contraindications.

- Accessible Resources: Provide readily accessible aromatherapy resources, such as essential oil libraries, guides, or expert consultations, to support employees in their wellness journey.

Conclusion: A Healthier, More Productive Workplace

Aromatherapy offers a holistic approach to addressing workplace stress and enhancing overall well-being. By incorporating essential oils into the work environment, employers can create a more pleasant and productive atmosphere that benefits both employees and the organization as a whole. As the use of aromatherapy in the workplace continues to grow, it demonstrates the commitment to employee wellness and the recognition of the powerful impact of a stress-free and invigorating work environment on job satisfaction and productivity.

The Art of Layering Essential Oils for a Lasting Scent

Introduction:

Creating a unique and long-lasting fragrance with essential oils is an art that allows you to customize scents that reflect your personality and preferences. One effective technique for achieving a lasting aroma is layering essential oils. In this comprehensive article, we will delve into the art of layering essential oils, exploring the science behind it, practical tips, and some enticing scent combinations to get you started.

Understanding the Basics:

Layering essential oils involves the strategic application of multiple oils to build a complex and harmonious scent profile. Each layer contributes to the overall aroma, and when done correctly, the result is a fragrance that lasts throughout the day.

The Science of Layering:

Layering works because essential oils have different volatilities, which determine how quickly they evaporate. Oils with lower volatilities evaporate slowly and serve as the base notes, while those with higher volatilities are the top notes that give the initial burst of scent. Middle notes bridge the gap between the two, providing balance and depth.

Building Your Fragrance:

1. Base Notes: Start with the base notes, which form the foundation of your scent. These oils are typically deep, warm, and earthy. Some popular base notes include:

- Sandalwood
- Patchouli
- Vetiver
- Cedarwood
- Frankincense

2. Middle Notes: Layer middle notes on top of the base to create complexity. These oils are often floral, herbal, or spicy. Examples of middle notes include:

- Lavender
- Rosemary
- Geranium
- Chamomile
- Ylang-ylang

3. Top Notes: Finally, add the top notes to provide an initial burst of scent. These oils are usually bright, fresh, and citrusy. Top note options include:

- Lemon
- Peppermint
- Bergamot
- Grapefruit
- Eucalyptus

Practical Layering Tips:

- Proper Dilution: Always dilute essential oils with a carrier oil before applying to the skin. This ensures safe use and helps the scent last longer.

- Layer on Pulse Points: Apply the layered blend to pulse points such as wrists, neck, and behind the ears. The warmth of these areas helps diffuse the scent throughout the day.

- Experiment: Don't be afraid to experiment with different combinations and ratios to find your perfect scent. Keep a journal to record your favorite blends.

- Wait Between Layers: Allow each layer to dry and settle before adding the next one. This prevents the scents from blending too quickly and allows you to appreciate each note.

Enticing Scent Combinations:

1. Citrus Burst:
   - Base: Cedarwood
   - Middle: Lavender
   - Top: Grapefruit

2. Earthy Elegance:
   - Base: Patchouli
   - Middle: Rosemary
   - Top: Bergamot

3. Floral Fantasy:
   - Base: Vetiver
   - Middle: Geranium
   - Top: Ylang-ylang

4. Minty Freshness:
   - Base: Sandalwood

- Middle: Chamomile

- Top: Peppermint

Conclusion: Personalized and Long-Lasting Fragrance

Layering essential oils is a creative and enjoyable way to craft a fragrance that is uniquely yours. By understanding the science behind layering and experimenting with various combinations, you can create scents that not only reflect your personality but also linger pleasantly throughout the day. Whether you're looking for a soothing blend to calm your senses or an invigorating mix to start your day with energy, layering essential oils offers a world of aromatic possibilities. So, embrace the art of layering and let your signature scent be an expression of your individuality.

Geranium Essential Oil: Balancing Emotions and Skin

Introduction:

Geranium essential oil, derived from the fragrant geranium plant, is a versatile and widely used essential oil known for its numerous therapeutic properties. This comprehensive article explores the diverse benefits of geranium essential oil, with a particular focus on its ability to balance emotions and support healthy skin.

The Essence of Geranium:

Geranium (Pelargonium graveolens) is a flowering plant native to South Africa. Its delicate pink to purple flowers emit a sweet, floral scent that is captured in the essential oil through steam distillation of the plant's leaves and stems. The oil is celebrated for its various chemical components, including geraniol and citronellol, which contribute to its distinct aroma and therapeutic effects.

Emotional Balance and Well-being:

One of the most remarkable aspects of geranium essential oil is its impact on emotional well-being. Here's how it helps in balancing emotions:

1. Elevates Mood: Geranium oil has mood-enhancing properties that can help alleviate feelings of stress, anxiety, and sadness. Its floral scent is often associated with positivity and emotional upliftment.

2. Stress Reduction: Inhaling geranium essential oil through diffusion or aromatherapy can reduce stress levels and promote relaxation. It has a calming effect on the nervous system, making it an excellent choice for relaxation routines.

3. Hormonal Balance: Geranium oil is particularly beneficial for women experiencing hormonal fluctuations. It can help ease symptoms of PMS and menopause, such as mood swings and irritability.

Skin Health and Beauty:

Geranium essential oil is equally renowned for its skin-nurturing properties. Whether used topically or in skincare products, it offers various advantages:

1. Balances Oily Skin: Geranium oil is known to regulate sebum production, making it ideal for those with oily or combination skin. It helps minimize excess oiliness and promotes a more balanced complexion.

2. Soothes Skin Irritations: The anti-inflammatory properties of geranium oil make it effective in soothing skin irritations like redness,

itching, and minor burns. It can be applied topically after dilution with a carrier oil.

3. Anti-Aging Benefits: Geranium oil's astringent qualities can help tighten the skin and reduce the appearance of wrinkles and fine lines. It is often incorporated into anti-aging skincare products.

4. Promotes Skin Healing: When diluted and applied to minor wounds or cuts, geranium essential oil can aid in the healing process by preventing infection and supporting tissue repair.

Practical Uses:

1. Aromatherapy: Diffuse geranium oil in your home or workspace to create a calming and uplifting atmosphere. It's an excellent choice for promoting emotional balance.

2. Skincare: Add a few drops of geranium oil to your daily moisturizer or create a customized facial oil blend to address specific skin concerns.

3. Massage: Diluted geranium oil can be used in massage therapy to relax muscles and soothe the mind. Its pleasant aroma enhances the massage experience.

Safety Considerations:

- Always dilute geranium essential oil with a carrier oil before applying it to the skin.

- Perform a patch test on a small area of skin to check for any allergic reactions.

- Consult a healthcare professional, especially during pregnancy or if you have specific medical conditions.

Conclusion: A Multifaceted Essential Oil

Geranium essential oil is a multifaceted gem that offers both emotional and skin-related benefits. Whether you seek to balance your mood, improve your skin's health, or simply enjoy its sweet, floral fragrance, geranium oil is a valuable addition to your aromatherapy and skincare routines. Harness its power to create emotional harmony and promote radiant, healthy skin.

Essential Oils for Eczema Relief: Soothing Inflamed Skin

Introduction:

Eczema, also known as atopic dermatitis, is a common skin condition characterized by redness, itching, and inflammation. While there is no cure for eczema, essential oils offer a natural and holistic approach to manage its symptoms and provide relief. In this comprehensive article, we'll explore how essential oils can be used effectively to soothe inflamed skin and alleviate the discomfort associated with eczema.

Understanding Eczema:

Eczema is a chronic skin condition that affects people of all ages. It often presents as dry, itchy, and inflamed patches of skin that can become red, scaly, and even painful. The exact cause of eczema is not fully understood, but it is believed to involve a combination of genetic, environmental, and immune system factors.

How Essential Oils Can Help:

Essential oils offer several benefits for eczema management:

1. Anti-Inflammatory Properties: Many essential oils have natural anti-inflammatory properties that can help reduce redness and swelling associated with eczema.

2. Moisturization: Eczema-prone skin tends to be dry and prone to moisture loss. Certain essential oils can help lock in moisture and prevent further dryness.

3. Relief from Itching: Essential oils can provide relief from the intense itching that often accompanies eczema, making it easier to resist scratching and further irritating the skin.

4. Antibacterial and Antifungal: Some essential oils possess antibacterial and antifungal properties, which can be beneficial in preventing secondary infections that may occur when the skin is broken from scratching.

Effective Essential Oils for Eczema:

1. Lavender Oil: Lavender oil is known for its anti-inflammatory and soothing properties. It can help reduce redness and itching, promoting a sense of calm.

2. Chamomile Oil: Chamomile is a gentle oil that can help soothe inflamed skin. It's particularly useful for eczema in children.

3. Tea Tree Oil: Tea tree oil has antibacterial and antifungal properties that can prevent infections in eczema-prone areas.

4. Frankincense Oil: Frankincense oil can help reduce inflammation and promote skin regeneration, making it suitable for eczema management.

5. Geranium Oil: Geranium oil is known for its skin-balancing properties, which can help with the dryness associated with eczema.

Safe Usage Tips:

- Always dilute essential oils with a carrier oil (such as jojoba, coconut, or almond oil) before applying them to the skin.
- Perform a patch test on a small area of skin to check for any allergic reactions or sensitivity.
- Use a small amount of the diluted oil and apply it gently to the affected area.

Practical Application:

1. Topical Application: Create a soothing blend by diluting a few drops of your chosen essential oil with a carrier oil. Apply it to the affected areas a few times a day.

2. Bath Soak: Add a few drops of essential oil to a warm bath to soothe widespread eczema symptoms.

3. Aromatherapy: Diffuse eczema-friendly essential oils in your home to create a calming and soothing atmosphere.

When to Consult a Professional:

While essential oils can provide relief for many eczema sufferers, it's important to consult a dermatologist or healthcare provider for severe or persistent cases. They can offer guidance on treatment options, including prescription medications or topical creams, to manage eczema effectively.

Conclusion: Natural Relief for Eczema

Eczema can be a challenging condition to manage, but essential oils can offer a natural and soothing approach to alleviate its symptoms. By incorporating the right essential oils into your skincare routine and following safe usage guidelines, you can find relief from itching, inflammation, and discomfort associated with eczema. Always consult with a healthcare professional for personalized advice on managing your eczema effectively.

The Psychological Impact of Essential Oils on Anxiety

Introduction:

Anxiety is a prevalent mental health concern that affects millions of people worldwide. While there are various treatments available, some individuals seek natural and complementary approaches to manage anxiety. Essential oils, derived from aromatic plants, have gained popularity for their potential psychological benefits in reducing anxiety. In this comprehensive article, we will explore the psychological impact of essential oils on anxiety, including how they work, popular choices, and practical usage.

Understanding Anxiety:

Anxiety is a complex emotional response characterized by excessive worry, fear, and a sense of impending danger or doom. It can manifest in various forms, including generalized anxiety disorder (GAD), social anxiety disorder, panic disorder, and specific phobias. Anxiety can significantly impact one's daily life, affecting relationships, work, and overall well-being.

How Essential Oils Can Help:

Essential oils offer a holistic and complementary approach to managing anxiety. While not a substitute for professional medical care, their aromatic compounds can influence the brain and nervous system, potentially alleviating anxiety symptoms. Here's how essential oils can help:

1. Aromatherapy: Aromatherapy involves inhaling the scent of essential oils. When inhaled, certain essential oils can interact with the olfactory system and influence brain regions responsible for emotions and stress responses.

2. Calming Effects: Many essential oils have natural calming properties that can promote relaxation, reduce stress, and create a sense of tranquility.

3. Stress Reduction: Inhaling specific essential oils can trigger the release of neurochemicals like serotonin and dopamine, which are associated with improved mood and reduced stress.

Popular Essential Oils for Anxiety:

1. Lavender Oil: Lavender is one of the most well-known essential oils for anxiety relief. Its soothing scent can help reduce feelings of nervousness and promote relaxation.

2. Chamomile Oil: Chamomile essential oil has anti-anxiety properties and can be especially helpful for calming the mind and improving sleep quality.

3. Frankincense Oil: Frankincense has a grounding aroma that can aid in reducing symptoms of anxiety and promoting a sense of emotional balance.

4. Ylang-Ylang Oil: Ylang-ylang is known for its ability to reduce stress and anxiety while promoting feelings of happiness and contentment.

5. Bergamot Oil: Bergamot essential oil has a citrusy scent that can lift mood and alleviate anxiety symptoms.

Practical Usage:

1. Diffusion: Use an essential oil diffuser to disperse the scent throughout your living space. Inhale the aroma regularly to experience its anxiety-reducing effects.

2. Topical Application: Dilute essential oils with a carrier oil (e.g., coconut or jojoba oil) and apply the mixture to pulse points, such as wrists and temples, for on-the-go anxiety relief.

3. Bath Soak: Add a few drops of anxiety-relieving essential oil to a warm bath for a relaxing soak.

4. Massage: Consider a calming aromatherapy massage using diluted essential oils to relax tense muscles and ease anxiety.

Safety Considerations:

- Perform a patch test before applying undiluted essential oils to your skin to check for allergic reactions.
- Consult a healthcare professional, especially if you are pregnant, nursing, or taking medications.

Conclusion: A Natural Approach to Anxiety Management

While essential oils may not be a standalone solution for anxiety disorders, they can be a valuable complement to traditional therapeutic approaches. The psychological impact of essential oils on anxiety is rooted in their ability to promote relaxation, reduce stress, and create a sense of emotional well-being. Whether through diffusion, topical application, or relaxation techniques, incorporating anxiety-relieving essential oils into your daily routine can offer a natural and aromatic path toward a calmer, more balanced state of mind.

Crafting Personalized Essential Oil Massage Blends

Introduction:

Massage therapy is a therapeutic practice that has been used for centuries to promote relaxation, alleviate tension, and enhance overall well-being. When combined with the power of essential oils, it becomes an even more potent tool for enhancing physical and emotional health. In this comprehensive article, we will explore the art of crafting personalized essential oil massage blends, including the benefits, considerations, and practical steps to create your own unique blends.

The Power of Massage and Essential Oils:

Massage therapy involves the manipulation of muscles and soft tissues to relieve tension, improve circulation, and promote relaxation. When essential oils are incorporated into massage, their aromatic compounds can enhance the therapeutic effects by:

1. Aromatherapy Benefits: Inhaling the scents of essential oils during a massage can influence emotions, reduce stress, and create a calming or invigorating atmosphere, depending on the chosen oils.

2. Skin Absorption: The skin can absorb essential oil molecules during massage, allowing their therapeutic properties to penetrate and benefit the body on a physical level.

3. Enhanced Relaxation: Essential oils can deepen the relaxation response, making massage sessions more effective in reducing muscle tension and mental stress.

Benefits of Personalized Blends:

Personalized essential oil massage blends offer several advantages:

1. Tailored to Individual Needs: You can create blends that address specific concerns, whether it's relaxation, pain relief, or emotional balance.

2. Enhanced Therapeutic Effects: Combining complementary essential oils can amplify their therapeutic properties and create a more holistic healing experience.

3. Unique Aromas: Crafting your blends allows you to explore various scents and customize the aroma to suit your preferences or your client's preferences.

Considerations Before Crafting Blends:

Before creating personalized massage blends, consider the following:

1. Individual Preferences: Determine the scents and effects that resonate with the person receiving the massage. Ask about any allergies or sensitivities.

2. Safety Precautions: Essential oils must be diluted with a carrier oil to avoid skin irritation. Ensure you're aware of any contraindications or safety concerns for specific oils.

3. Therapeutic Goals: Define the purpose of the massage. Are you aiming for relaxation, pain relief, or emotional support? This will guide your essential oil selection.

Practical Steps to Crafting Blends:

1. Choose Your Base Oil: Start with a carrier oil like jojoba, sweet almond, or coconut oil. These oils dilute essential oils and provide a smooth glide during the massage.

2. Select Your Essential Oils: Based on the therapeutic goals and preferences, choose two to three essential oils that complement each other. For relaxation, consider lavender, chamomile, and frankincense. For pain relief, try peppermint, eucalyptus, and ginger.

3. Dilution Ratio: A typical dilution ratio is 2-3% essential oil to carrier oil. For example, for every 10ml of carrier oil, add 3-6 drops of essential oil.

4. Blending: Combine the chosen essential oils with the carrier oil in a glass bottle. Start with a smaller amount of essential oil, as you can always add more if needed.

5. Patch Test: Perform a patch test on a small area of skin to ensure there are no adverse reactions or allergies.

6. Adjustments: If the blend is too strong or weak, adjust the essential oil quantity accordingly. Keep notes of your blends for future reference.

Conclusion: The Art of Healing Touch and Aroma

Crafting personalized essential oil massage blends allows you to harness the combined therapeutic power of touch and aroma. By selecting the right essential oils, diluting them properly, and tailoring the experience to individual needs, you can create a truly unique and effective massage blend. Whether you're a massage therapist or someone looking to enhance your self-care routine, the art of crafting personalized massage blends can add a new dimension of healing and relaxation to your practice.

Ylang-Ylang Essential Oil: Sensual and Calming Properties

Introduction:

Ylang-ylang essential oil, derived from the blossoms of the Cananga odorata tree native to Southeast Asia, is a fragrant and versatile oil known for its exotic aroma and numerous therapeutic benefits. Renowned for its sensual and calming properties, ylang-ylang has been used for centuries in traditional medicine, aromatherapy, and perfumery. In this comprehensive article, we will explore the origins, composition, and various uses of ylang-ylang essential oil, shedding light on its unique characteristics and the ways it can enhance your well-being.

Origins and Extraction:

Ylang-ylang, often referred to as the "flower of flowers," is native to countries like Indonesia, Malaysia, and the Philippines. The essential oil is extracted through steam distillation of the vibrant, star-shaped flowers of the ylang-ylang tree. Depending on the distillation process and timing, different grades of ylang-ylang oil are produced, each with its distinct aroma and properties.

Composition of Ylang-Ylang Essential Oil:

Ylang-ylang essential oil contains a rich array of chemical compounds that contribute to its therapeutic effects. Key constituents include:

1. Linalool: Known for its calming and soothing properties, linalool helps reduce stress and anxiety.

2. Geranyl acetate: This compound imparts ylang-ylang's characteristic floral aroma and contributes to its sedative effects.

3. Beta-caryophyllene: Exhibiting anti-inflammatory properties, this compound can help soothe irritated skin.

4. Methyl benzoate: Known for its pleasant aroma, methyl benzoate contributes to ylang-ylang's sweet scent.

Sensual and Calming Properties:

Ylang-ylang essential oil is celebrated for its sensual and calming properties, making it a popular choice for various applications:

1. Aphrodisiac: Ylang-ylang is often considered an aphrodisiac due to its ability to enhance sensuality and intimacy. Its exotic floral scent can set the mood for romance and passion.

2. Emotional Balance: Ylang-ylang is known to promote emotional balance by reducing feelings of anxiety, stress, and tension. It has a calming effect on the mind and can help alleviate symptoms of mild depression.

3. Sleep Aid: Diffusing ylang-ylang essential oil before bedtime can promote relaxation and improve sleep quality. It helps create a serene and peaceful atmosphere.

4. Skin and Hair Care: Ylang-ylang oil can be added to skincare products to help balance oily skin and promote a healthy complexion. It is also used in hair treatments to nourish and add shine.

Practical Uses:

1. Aromatherapy: Add a few drops of ylang-ylang oil to a diffuser to create a soothing and sensual atmosphere in your home.

2. Massage: Dilute ylang-ylang with a carrier oil and use it in a sensual massage to relax muscles and enhance intimacy.

3. Bath Soak: Mix a few drops of ylang-ylang oil with Epsom salts and add to a warm bath for a luxurious and calming soak.

4. Skincare: Incorporate ylang-ylang oil into your skincare routine by adding a drop or two to your moisturizer or facial serum.

Safety Precautions:

While ylang-ylang is generally safe for topical and aromatic use, it's important to consider individual sensitivities. Always perform a patch test and dilute it with a carrier oil before applying it to the skin. Avoid using excessive amounts, as its potent scent can become overwhelming.

Conclusion: Aromatic Elegance and Tranquility

Ylang-ylang essential oil, with its sensual and calming properties, is a valuable addition to the world of aromatherapy and natural wellness. Whether you seek to enhance your emotional well-being, promote intimacy, or create a serene environment, ylang-ylang's exotic and elegant aroma can uplift your spirits and bring tranquility to your life. Explore the many facets of this remarkable oil and unlock its potential to enhance your physical and emotional health.

Essential Oils for Coping with Grief and Loss

Introduction:

Grief and loss are universal human experiences, and the emotional toll they can take on individuals is profound. While there is no magic solution for healing from grief, many people turn to complementary and holistic approaches to ease the emotional burden. Essential oils, derived from aromatic plants, have gained recognition for their potential therapeutic benefits in helping individuals cope with grief and loss. In this comprehensive article, we will explore the use of essential oils as a supportive tool in the grieving process, including their emotional effects, application methods, and the importance of self-care during times of loss.

Understanding Grief and Loss:

Grief is a complex emotional response to loss, which can result from various life events, including the death of a loved one, the end of a relationship, or significant life changes. It encompasses a range of emotions, from sadness and anger to guilt and confusion. Grief is a highly individual process, and there is no right or wrong way to experience it.

How Essential Oils Can Help:

Essential oils offer a holistic approach to emotional support during times of grief and loss. While they are not a substitute for professional counseling or therapy, their aromatic compounds can influence the limbic system, which is responsible for emotions and memory. Here's how essential oils can assist in coping with grief:

1. Emotional Comfort: Many essential oils have calming and soothing properties that can help ease emotional distress and promote relaxation.

2. Mind-Body Connection: Inhaling certain essential oils can trigger the release of neurotransmitters like serotonin and dopamine, which are associated with improved mood and emotional balance.

3. Self-Care Ritual: Using essential oils in self-care routines can provide moments of solace and reflection, allowing individuals to process their emotions.

Popular Essential Oils for Grief and Loss:

1. Lavender Oil: Lavender is known for its calming and soothing properties, making it an excellent choice for reducing anxiety and promoting relaxation during moments of grief.

2. Frankincense Oil: Frankincense has a grounding aroma that can provide emotional support, helping individuals find inner peace and acceptance.

3. Rose Oil: Rose essential oil is associated with love and compassion. Its sweet and comforting scent can provide solace and aid in emotional healing.

4. Bergamot Oil: Bergamot's citrusy aroma can lift mood and provide a sense of hope during times of sadness.

5. Chamomile Oil: Chamomile essential oil is gentle and can help reduce feelings of anger and irritability often associated with grief.

Practical Application Methods:

1. Aromatherapy: Use a diffuser to disperse the scent of essential oils in your living space, creating a comforting and tranquil atmosphere.

2. Topical Application: Dilute essential oils with a carrier oil and apply the mixture to pulse points, such as wrists and temples, for on-the-go emotional support.

3. Bath Soak: Add a few drops of essential oil to a warm bath for a soothing and calming experience.

4. Inhalation: Inhale the aroma of essential oils from a tissue or inhale directly from the bottle when needed.

The Importance of Self-Care:

Coping with grief and loss is emotionally draining, and self-care becomes paramount during this time. Essential oils can be a part of a broader self-care routine that includes practices such as meditation, journaling, seeking support from loved ones, and professional counseling or therapy.

Conclusion: A Fragrant Path to Healing

While essential oils cannot erase the pain of grief and loss, they can serve as a supportive tool in the healing process. The emotional comfort and solace that essential oils offer can provide moments of respite and emotional release during difficult times. By incorporating essential oils into self-care routines and seeking support when needed, individuals can navigate the challenging journey of grief with greater emotional resilience and self-compassion.

The Use of Essential Oils in Shamanic Practices

Introduction:

Shamanism is an ancient spiritual and healing practice that has been used by indigenous cultures worldwide for millennia. It involves connecting with the spirit world, facilitating healing, and seeking guidance through various rituals and ceremonies. Essential oils, with their potent aromatic and therapeutic properties, have played a significant role in shamanic practices. In this comprehensive article, we will delve into the history, significance, and practical applications of essential oils in the context of shamanic traditions, exploring how these natural substances enhance spiritual experiences and healing.

The History and Significance:

Essential oils have been an integral part of shamanic rituals and healing ceremonies for centuries. These natural extracts, obtained from aromatic plants, were revered for their ability to:

1. Alter Consciousness: Certain essential oils have psychoactive properties that can induce altered states of consciousness, which are often essential for shamanic journeys and visions.

2. Evoke Spiritual Connection: The fragrant scents of essential oils were believed to bridge the physical and spiritual realms, making it easier for shamans to communicate with the spirit world.

3. Facilitate Healing: Essential oils were used to cleanse, purify, and protect individuals during rituals, as well as to aid in physical and emotional healing.

Practical Applications in Shamanic Practices:

1. Anointing: Shamans would anoint themselves and others with essential oils before and during ceremonies. Oils like frankincense, myrrh, and cedarwood were common choices for their grounding and spiritually uplifting properties.

2. Smudging: Essential oils were often added to smudging bundles, enhancing the cleansing and purifying effects of the ritual. Sage, cedar, and palo santo essential oils were favored for this purpose.

3. Aromatherapy: Inhaling the scent of specific essential oils, either through diffusion or direct inhalation, could induce trance-like states or heightened spiritual awareness. Oils like lavender, pine, and patchouli were used for their aromatic influence on mood and perception.

4. Spiritual Protection: Essential oils with protective properties, such as juniper, myrrh, and rosemary, were used to create barriers against negative energies and entities during shamanic journeys.

5. Psychopomp Work: Shamans often assisted spirits in transitioning to the afterlife. Essential oils like rose, sandalwood, and lavender were used to create a peaceful and loving environment for this work.

Modern Interpretations:

In contemporary shamanic practices, essential oils are still valued for their ability to deepen spiritual experiences, promote healing, and support emotional well-being. While traditional methods remain relevant, modern practitioners have developed new ways to incorporate essential oils into their rituals:

1. Diffusion: Using essential oil diffusers, practitioners can infuse their ceremonial spaces with the scent of sacred oils, creating a conducive atmosphere for journeying and meditation.

2. Personal Blends: Shamans and modern practitioners often create personalized essential oil blends that resonate with their intentions and the energy of their work.

3. Cleansing and Clearing: Essential oils are used to cleanse and clear energy in spaces, objects, and the self before, during, and after shamanic work.

4. Integration with Other Modalities: Essential oils can be integrated with other shamanic practices, such as sound healing, crystal work, and plant medicine ceremonies.

Conclusion: Ancestral Wisdom Meets Modern Healing

The use of essential oils in shamanic practices is a testament to the enduring wisdom of indigenous cultures and their profound understanding of the natural world. Whether in traditional rituals or contemporary ceremonies, essential oils continue to play a vital role in connecting individuals with the spirit realm, facilitating healing, and promoting spiritual growth. As more people seek holistic and spiritually enriching experiences, the integration of essential oils into shamanic practices remains a powerful and resonant path to inner exploration and transformation.

Myrtle Essential Oil: A Symbol of Love and Healing

Introduction:

Myrtle essential oil, derived from the aromatic myrtle plant, holds a special place in history and mythology as a symbol of love, healing, and renewal. This versatile oil boasts a range of therapeutic properties, from promoting emotional balance to supporting physical well-being. In this comprehensive article, we will explore the history, properties, uses, and symbolism of myrtle essential oil, shedding light on its rich cultural heritage and its relevance in contemporary aromatherapy and wellness.

Botanical Origins:

Myrtle (Myrtus communis) is a small evergreen shrub native to the Mediterranean region. It has glossy green leaves, fragrant white flowers, and small blue-black berries. The essential oil is obtained through steam distillation of the plant's leaves, twigs, and flowers.

Historical Significance:

Myrtle has a long and storied history dating back to ancient civilizations. Some notable mentions include:

1. Ancient Greece: Myrtle was sacred to Aphrodite, the Greek goddess of love and beauty. It was used in wedding ceremonies and to adorn bridal bouquets as a symbol of love and fertility.

2. Ancient Rome: In Roman mythology, Venus, the goddess of love, was associated with myrtle. Myrtle wreaths were worn by brides and used to decorate homes during festivals.

3. Judaism: Myrtle is one of the Four Species used during the Jewish holiday of Sukkot, symbolizing renewal and growth.

4. Medicinal Use: Throughout history, myrtle has been valued for its medicinal properties, including its role in supporting respiratory health and promoting emotional well-being.

Therapeutic Properties:

Myrtle essential oil is prized for its numerous therapeutic qualities:

1. Emotional Balance: Myrtle oil is known for its calming and uplifting properties, making it an effective choice for reducing stress, anxiety, and feelings of sadness.

2. Respiratory Support: It has been used to alleviate respiratory issues, such as coughs, congestion, and asthma, thanks to its mucolytic and expectorant properties.

3. Antiseptic: Myrtle essential oil possesses antiseptic and antibacterial properties, making it useful for skin and wound care.

4. Astringent: It can be used to improve the appearance of oily or acne-prone skin and tighten pores.

Modern Uses:

1. Aromatherapy: Myrtle oil is a popular choice in aromatherapy to promote emotional balance, relaxation, and mental clarity. Diffusing it can create a tranquil atmosphere.

2. Skincare: It can be added to skincare products to improve the appearance of blemishes, oily skin, and minor skin irritations.

3. Respiratory Support: Myrtle oil can be blended with a carrier oil and applied topically to the chest or used in steam inhalation to ease respiratory discomfort.

4. Massage: Incorporating myrtle oil into massage blends can enhance relaxation and soothe muscle tension.

Symbolism and Folklore:

Myrtle has symbolized love, purity, and renewal across various cultures. In addition to its association with Aphrodite and Venus, it has been linked to:

1. Marriage and Fidelity: Myrtle is often used in weddings and bridal bouquets as a symbol of love, commitment, and marital bliss.

2. Healing and Protection: It has been used as a protective charm and an emblem of healing, representing physical and emotional rejuvenation.

3. Renewal and Growth: Myrtle's evergreen nature and ability to regenerate symbolize renewal, growth, and the cycles of life.

Conclusion: A Time-Honored Elixir

Myrtle essential oil, with its rich history and diverse therapeutic properties, continues to be a cherished botanical treasure in the world of aromatherapy and holistic wellness. Whether you are seeking emotional balance, respiratory support, or simply a fragrant reminder of love and renewal, myrtle essential oil offers a time-honored elixir that connects us to ancient traditions and the enduring power of nature's gifts. Its soothing aroma and versatile applications make it a valuable addition to your essential oil collection and a symbol of love, healing, and hope.

Essential Oils for Healthy Hair and Scalp: DIY Treatments

Introduction:

Achieving and maintaining healthy hair and scalp is a common goal for many people. Essential oils, with their natural and therapeutic properties, offer a holistic approach to hair care. In this comprehensive article, we will explore how essential oils can benefit your hair and scalp, discuss the best essential oils for various hair concerns, and provide DIY treatments to promote luscious locks and a healthy scalp.

Understanding Hair and Scalp Health:

Before delving into the world of essential oils, it's essential to understand the basics of hair and scalp health:

1. Hair Structure: Hair consists of a protein called keratin. The hair shaft extends from the follicle, which is embedded in the scalp.

2. Scalp Health: A healthy scalp is crucial for healthy hair growth. It provides the necessary environment for hair follicles to thrive.

Benefits of Essential Oils for Hair and Scalp:

Essential oils offer a range of benefits for your hair and scalp, including:

1. Promoting Hair Growth: Some essential oils stimulate hair follicles, encouraging hair growth and reducing hair loss.

2. Balancing Scalp: Essential oils can help maintain a balanced and moisturized scalp, reducing dandruff and itchiness.

3. Strengthening Hair: Certain oils can strengthen hair strands, reducing breakage and split ends.

4. Enhancing Shine: Essential oils can add shine and luster to your hair, making it look healthy and vibrant.

Top Essential Oils for Hair and Scalp:

1. Lavender Oil: Promotes hair growth, balances scalp oil production, and has a calming scent.

2. Rosemary Oil: Stimulates hair follicles, improves circulation, and strengthens hair.

3. Peppermint Oil: Refreshes the scalp, improves hair thickness, and reduces dandruff.

4. Tea Tree Oil: Has antifungal properties, making it effective against dandruff and scalp irritation.

5. Lemon Oil: Adds shine to hair, clarifies the scalp, and has a refreshing scent.

DIY Essential Oil Hair Treatments:

1. Nourishing Hair Mask:

- Ingredients: 2 tbsp coconut oil, 3-5 drops lavender oil, 3-5 drops rosemary oil.

- Instructions: Mix ingredients, apply to damp hair, leave for 30 minutes, and rinse.

2. Scalp Massage Oil:

- Ingredients: 2 tbsp jojoba oil, 3-5 drops tea tree oil, 3-5 drops peppermint oil.

- Instructions: Massage into the scalp, leave for 15-30 minutes, and shampoo.

3. Dandruff Treatment:

- Ingredients: 2 tbsp apple cider vinegar, 3-5 drops tea tree oil, 3-5 drops lemon oil.
- Instructions: Mix, apply to the scalp, leave for 20 minutes, and rinse.

4. Hair Growth Serum:

- Ingredients: 2 tbsp argan oil, 3-5 drops rosemary oil, 3-5 drops lavender oil.
- Instructions: Apply to the scalp daily, massage gently, and leave overnight.

5. Shine-Boosting Rinse:

- Ingredients: 1 cup water, 3-5 drops lemon oil.
- Instructions: Mix, use as a final rinse after shampooing, and don't rinse afterward.

Tips for Safe Use:

- Always dilute essential oils with a carrier oil to prevent skin and scalp irritation.
- Do a patch test before applying any new oil blend to your scalp to ensure you're not allergic or sensitive.
- Use essential oils sparingly; a few drops are usually sufficient.
- Consult with a healthcare professional if you have any underlying scalp conditions.

Conclusion: Beautiful Hair, Naturally

Essential oils offer a natural and effective way to support the health of your hair and scalp. Whether you're looking to stimulate hair growth, combat dandruff, or simply enhance the overall condition of your locks, essential oils can be a valuable addition to your hair care routine. Experiment with different oils and DIY treatments to discover what works best for your unique hair and scalp needs. With regular care and the power of essential oils, you can enjoy healthy, vibrant hair that shines with natural beauty.

The Art of Aromachology: How Scents Influence Behavior

Introduction:

The power of scent is a fascinating and often underestimated aspect of human experience. Aromachology, the study of how scents influence behavior, emotions, and psychological well-being, sheds light on the profound impact that fragrances have on our lives. This comprehensive article explores the art of aromachology, delving into the science behind scent perception, the psychology of fragrance, and practical applications for enhancing various aspects of our daily lives.

The Science of Scent Perception:

1. Olfactory System: Our sense of smell, or olfaction, is a complex and highly sensitive sensory system. The olfactory bulb, located in the brain, plays a central role in processing scent information.

2. Scent Molecules: When we encounter a fragrance, scent molecules are released into the air and inhaled through our nose. These molecules bind to receptors in the olfactory bulb, sending signals to the brain.

3. Emotional Center: The olfactory bulb is closely connected to the brain's emotional center, the limbic system. This link explains why scents can evoke strong emotional responses.

The Psychology of Fragrance:

1. Emotion and Memory: Scent has a remarkable ability to trigger memories and emotions. Certain scents can transport us back in time, evoking nostalgia, comfort, or happiness.

2. Mood Enhancement: Fragrances can influence mood. Citrus scents, for example, are often associated with feelings of energy and positivity, while lavender is known for its calming effects.

3. Stress Reduction: Aromatherapy, a branch of aromachology, uses scents like lavender, chamomile, and rose to reduce stress and anxiety.

4. Behavioral Responses: Scents can influence behavior. The smell of freshly baked bread in a bakery can entice customers to make a purchase, while a calming scent in a spa can encourage relaxation.

Practical Applications of Aromachology:

1. Home and Environment: Choose scents that align with the desired ambiance of a space. Peppermint may boost alertness in a home office, while lavender can promote relaxation in a bedroom.

2. Product Development: Perfumers and product developers use aromachology to create scents that enhance the appeal of products, from cosmetics to cleaning agents.

3. Marketing and Retail: Retailers strategically use scents to influence customer behavior. A pleasant store fragrance can encourage longer visits and increased spending.

4. Therapeutic Use: Aromatherapists use specific scents to address various physical and emotional concerns, such as headaches, insomnia, or stress management.

Common Scents and Their Effects:

1. Lavender: Known for its calming properties, lavender is often used to reduce anxiety and improve sleep quality.

2. Citrus: Scents like lemon, orange, and grapefruit are invigorating and can boost mood and energy levels.

3. Rose: Rose is associated with romance and can evoke feelings of love and sensuality.

4. Peppermint: Refreshing and stimulating, peppermint can enhance alertness and concentration.

5. Vanilla: Warm and comforting, vanilla is often used to create a cozy and inviting atmosphere.

The Art of Personalized Fragrance:

1. Signature Scent: Many people have a signature scent, a fragrance that reflects their personality and becomes part of their identity.

2. Creating Mood: Individuals can choose fragrances that align with their goals and emotions for the day, whether it's focus, relaxation, or motivation.

3. Personal Rituals: Incorporating scent into personal rituals, such as applying a favorite perfume or lighting scented candles, can enhance mindfulness and well-being.

Conclusion: Scent as a Powerful Ally

Aromachology reminds us that the world of fragrance is not only about smelling pleasant scents but also about harnessing their potential to enhance our lives. By understanding the science and psychology of scent, we can make intentional choices about the fragrances we surround ourselves with, whether it's to create a calming home environment, boost productivity at work, or simply enjoy the myriad sensory pleasures that the world of scent offers. As we navigate the art of aromachology, we discover that fragrance is a powerful ally in shaping our experiences, emotions, and behaviors, enriching our lives in countless ways.

Combining Yoga and Aromatherapy for Mind-Body Balance

Introduction:

Yoga and aromatherapy are two holistic practices that, when combined, create a powerful synergy for achieving mind-body balance and overall well-being. This comprehensive article explores the art of combining yoga and aromatherapy, shedding light on the benefits, techniques, and considerations for integrating these practices into your wellness routine.

Understanding Yoga and Aromatherapy:

1. Yoga: Yoga is an ancient practice that combines physical ures (asanas), breath control (pranayama), and meditation to promote physical, mental, and spiritual harmony.

2. Aromatherapy: Aromatherapy is the use of aromatic essential oils derived from plants to enhance physical and emotional well-being. These oils are often used in massages, diffusers, or as topical applications.

The Benefits of Combining Yoga and Aromatherapy:

1. Enhanced Relaxation: Aromatherapy can deepen the relaxation achieved during yoga practice, allowing you to release physical and mental tension more effectively.

2. Emotional Support: Certain essential oils can help address specific emotional states, such as lavender for calmness or citrus oils for upliftment, enhancing the emotional aspect of yoga.

3. Mindful Practice: Aromatherapy encourages mindfulness during yoga, as you focus on the scents and sensations, deepening your mind-body connection.

4. Stress Reduction: Combining yoga's stress-reducing benefits with aromatherapy's calming scents can be particularly effective for managing stress and anxiety.

Practical Techniques for Combining Yoga and Aromatherapy:

1. Diffusion: Use an essential oil diffuser in your yoga space to infuse the air with calming scents before and during your practice.

2. Topical Application: Dilute essential oils with a carrier oil and apply them to pulse points, such as wrists and temples, before beginning your practice.

3. Yoga Mat Spray: Create a DIY yoga mat spray by mixing water and a few drops of essential oil to refresh your mat and create a pleasant practice environment.

4. Aromatherapy During Savasana: Place a drop of calming essential oil on a tissue and tuck it under your yoga mat during savasana (final relaxation) for a soothing experience.

Best Essential Oils for Yoga:

1. Lavender: Calming and grounding, lavender oil can enhance relaxation during restorative or yin yoga practices.

2. Frankincense: Elevating and spiritually grounding, frankincense is ideal for enhancing meditation and deepening your yoga practice.

3. Peppermint: Invigorating and refreshing, peppermint oil can be used to energize and awaken your senses during dynamic yoga styles.

4. Eucalyptus: Clearing and refreshing, eucalyptus can support focused breathing during pranayama and enhance your overall practice.

Considerations and Safety:

- Always dilute essential oils properly to avoid skin irritation.
- Choose high-quality, pure essential oils from reputable sources.
- Be mindful of any allergies or sensitivities you may have to specific scents.
- Consult with a healthcare professional if you have any underlying health conditions.

Conclusion: A Harmonious Blend

Combining yoga and aromatherapy creates a harmonious blend of ancient practices that nourish the mind, body, and spirit. By integrating the healing power of scent into your yoga practice, you can deepen your connection to your inner self, enhance relaxation, and elevate the overall experience. Whether you're a seasoned yogi or just beginning your yoga journey, exploring the world of yoga and aromatherapy can lead to greater balance and well-being, enriching your holistic approach to health and self-care.

Essential Oils for Pet Anxiety: Calming Furry Friends

Introduction:

Just like humans, pets can experience anxiety and stress in various situations. Whether it's thunderstorms, separation anxiety, or visits to the vet, dealing with a distressed pet can be challenging. This comprehensive article explores the use of essential oils to help alleviate pet anxiety, offering natural and holistic solutions for calming your furry friends.

Understanding Pet Anxiety:

1. Causes of Anxiety: Pet anxiety can be triggered by a range of factors, including loud noises (thunder, fireworks), separation from their owner, car rides, or new environments.

2. Symptoms: Signs of pet anxiety can vary but may include restlessness, pacing, panting, hiding, excessive barking, or destructive behavior.

3. Holistic Approach: Essential oils provide a holistic approach to managing pet anxiety, focusing on their emotional well-being.

Safe Use of Essential Oils for Pets:

1. Dilution: Essential oils must always be diluted with a carrier oil before applying them to pets. The dilution ratio should be much lower than for humans.

2. Application: Apply the diluted oil to areas where your pet can't lick it off, such as the back of the neck or the base of the tail.

3. Observation: Monitor your pet's reaction when introducing them to essential oils. If they show signs of discomfort, discontinue use.

Top Essential Oils for Pet Anxiety:

1. Lavender: Lavender oil is renowned for its calming properties and can help reduce anxiety in pets. It's particularly useful for situations like thunderstorms or car rides.

2. Chamomile: Chamomile oil has soothing and anti-anxiety effects. It's gentle on pets and can be used to calm nerves.

3. Frankincense: Frankincense oil promotes relaxation and can help ease your pet's anxiety during stressful situations.

4. Valerian: Valerian oil has sedative properties and can be used sparingly to alleviate anxiety in pets.

Ways to Use Essential Oils for Pet Anxiety:

1. Diffusion: Use an essential oil diffuser to disperse calming scents throughout your home, creating a soothing environment for your pet.

2. Pet-Friendly Sprays: Some companies offer pet-specific essential oil sprays designed to reduce anxiety. These can be sprayed on their bedding or in their living space.

3. Massage: Gently massage a diluted essential oil blend onto your pet's neck or back to promote relaxation.

4. Aromatherapy Jewelry: Some pet collars or tags come with small compartments where you can place a few drops of essential oil for your pet to inhale.

Considerations and Safety:

- Consult with your veterinarian before using essential oils on your pet, especially if they have underlying health conditions or are pregnant.
- Avoid using essential oils on cats, as they can be more sensitive to certain oils. Always consult with a vet when considering essential oil use for cats.

- Store essential oils out of your pet's reach to prevent accidental ingestion.

Conclusion: A Calmer, Happier Pet

Pet anxiety can be distressing for both you and your furry friend, but with the right approach, you can help them find peace and comfort. Essential oils offer a natural and gentle way to alleviate pet anxiety and create a soothing atmosphere in your home. By using essential oils safely and in consultation with your veterinarian, you can help your pet lead a calmer and happier life, free from the burdens of anxiety and stress.

The Environmental Impact of Essential Oil Production

Introduction:

Essential oils have gained immense popularity for their therapeutic and aromatic qualities, but their production can have significant environmental implications. This educational article explores the environmental impact of essential oil production, shedding light on the factors contributing to both positive and negative effects on the environment.

Positive Environmental Aspects:

1. Sustainable Farming Practices: Many essential oil producers have adopted sustainable farming practices that prioritize soil health, reduce pesticide use, and promote biodiversity. This approach minimizes soil degradation and benefits local ecosystems.

2. Wildcrafting: Some essential oils are obtained through wildcrafting, which involves harvesting plants from their natural habitat. When done responsibly, wildcrafting can support the conservation of native species and habitats.

3. Certified Organic Production: Organic essential oil production prohibits the use of synthetic pesticides and fertilizers, promoting healthier ecosystems and reducing chemical pollution.

Negative Environmental Aspects:

1. Deforestation: In some regions, essential oil production has contributed to deforestation as forests are cleared to make way for commercial plantations. This can result in habitat loss for wildlife and disrupt local ecosystems.

2. Monoculture Plantations: Large-scale essential oil production often relies on monoculture plantations, where a single crop is grown over extensive areas. Monocultures can deplete soil nutrients, increase susceptibility to pests, and reduce biodiversity.

3. Water Consumption: The extraction of essential oils can be water-intensive. In regions with water scarcity, excessive water use can strain local water resources.

Chemical Usage: The use of synthetic pesticides and herbicides in conventional essential oil production can lead to chemical pollution, harming both the environment and nearby communities.

Air Pollution: Certain extraction methods, such as steam distillation, can release volatile organic compounds (VOCs) into the air, contributing to air pollution.

Waste Generation: The extraction process generates waste, such as plant material or spent biomass. Improper disposal of this waste can have negative environmental consequences.

Transportation: The global distribution of essential oils involves transportation, which contributes to greenhouse gas emissions and air pollution.

Environmental Conservation Efforts:

1. Certifications: Look for essential oils with certifications like "USDA Organic" or "Fair Trade" to support environmentally friendly and socially responsible practices.

2. Sustainable Sourcing: Choose essential oil brands that prioritize sustainable sourcing and support efforts to protect natural habitats.

3. Local and Small-Scale Producers: Supporting local and small-scale essential oil producers often aligns with more environmentally friendly practices.

Conclusion: Balancing Aromatherapy and Environmental Responsibility

As consumers, our choices can influence the environmental impact of essential oil production. By selecting products from companies committed to sustainable and responsible practices, we can contribute to positive change. Additionally, being mindful of our own essential oil usage, minimizing waste, and reducing overconsumption can help strike a balance between enjoying the benefits of aromatherapy and being environmentally responsible. Ultimately, it is our collective responsibility to protect the planet while enjoying the therapeutic benefits of essential oils.

Mindful Blending: The Art of Creating Harmonious Essential Oil Combinations

Introduction:

Aromatherapy, the art of using essential oils for therapeutic and emotional benefits, often involves the careful blending of different oils. Creating harmonious essential oil combinations is both a science and an art, requiring an understanding of each oil's properties and an appreciation for the resulting synergy. In this comprehensive article, we explore the principles and techniques of mindful blending to help you craft personalized, effective, and balanced essential oil blends.

Understanding Essential Oil Properties:

1. Base Notes: These oils are typically grounding, with deep, long-lasting scents. Examples include cedarwood, patchouli, and vetiver.

2. Middle Notes: These oils serve as the heart of the blend, often balancing between top and base notes. Lavender, rosemary, and geranium are common middle notes.

3. Top Notes: These oils have light, uplifting scents that evaporate quickly. They provide the initial fragrance but dissipate sooner. Examples include citrus oils like lemon, orange, and bergamot.

4. Note Intensity: Consider the relative strength of each oil's scent, as it can influence the overall aroma of your blend.

Balancing the Aroma:

1. The Rule of Thirds: A classic blending technique involves using one-third top notes, one-third middle notes, and one-third base notes to create a balanced aroma.

2. Personal Preferences: Recognize that individual preferences play a significant role in blending. What may be harmonious to one person may not be to another.

Creating a Theme or Purpose:

1. Therapeutic Goals: Identify the specific therapeutic goals you want to achieve with your blend, such as relaxation, focus, or immune support.

2. Emotional Impact: Essential oils can influence emotions. Consider the emotional impact you want your blend to have, whether it's calming, uplifting, or grounding.

Blending Techniques:

1. Layering: Begin with a base note, add a middle note, and finish with a top note. This sequential layering can help achieve balance.

2. Dilution: Always dilute essential oils with a carrier oil to ensure safety and prevent skin irritation.

3. Scent Testing: Blend small amounts of oils on a scent strip or your skin to gauge how they interact before creating a larger batch.

Sample Essential Oil Blends:

1. Calming Blend: Lavender (middle note), cedarwood (base note), and bergamot (top note) for relaxation and stress relief.

2. Energizing Blend: Peppermint (top note), rosemary (middle note), and vetiver (base note) for a refreshing and invigorating scent.

3. Balancing Blend: Geranium (middle note), frankincense (base note), and lemon (top note) for emotional balance and focus.

Conclusion: Crafting Your Signature Scents

Mindful blending of essential oils is a deeply rewarding and creative process. Whether you're creating blends for aromatherapy, massage, or personal fragrances, the principles of balance, purpose, and understanding oil properties will guide you toward harmonious combinations. Remember to document your recipes, experiment, and trust your intuition. With practice and mindfulness, you can develop your unique approach to creating essential oil blends that enhance your well-being and delight your senses.

Conclusion

Congratulations, you've just unlocked the door to a world of essential oils knowledge that will serve you well for years to come. This book isn't just a one-time read; it's your trusty companion, a quick reference, and a source of inspiration whenever you need it.

As you continue your journey with essential oils, remember that you now possess a solid foundation. You can confidently explore the aromatic wonders, share your insights with others, and craft blends that cater to your unique needs.

Whether you're using essential oils for personal wellness, expanding your business, or simply nurturing a passion, you're on a path filled with endless possibilities. The wisdom you've gained here will be your guide, helping you make informed decisions and achieve your goals.

We wish you boundless success in your endeavors with essential oils. May your aromatic adventures be enriching, your blends be harmonious, and your well-being be ever enhanced. Cheers to your journey, and may it be filled with aromatic delights and positive transformations.

About the Author

Sydney Brown has spent over thirty-five years in the business world and later in the corporate world. She has learned what works and what doesn't when the goal is to get out of the stale, vanilla world of the generations before us.

She believes that each person has at least one successful business, one book, and one grand adventure in them, but most people don't know how to figure out their best fit, so they stay where they are.

She is a best-selling author, speaker, and coach, helping people reach out of their current situation and reinvent themselves so they can do more than exist and survive while in this great space.

Personally, she's a mom of two adulting children and proudly owns the title of "Crazy Cat Lady" among her friends. After too many years of avoiding living life, she is on a mission to help others identify and begin their own "Great Ascension."

Let's Connect

If you've enjoyed this book, you'll love what else is ahead!

Start out at https://beyourownsolution.com/ and see what you can look forward to.

We have courses, certifications, and life and business focused free groups!

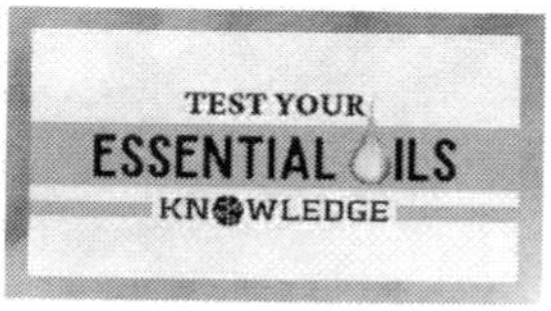

Free Essential Oil Quiz

Click to Sign Up

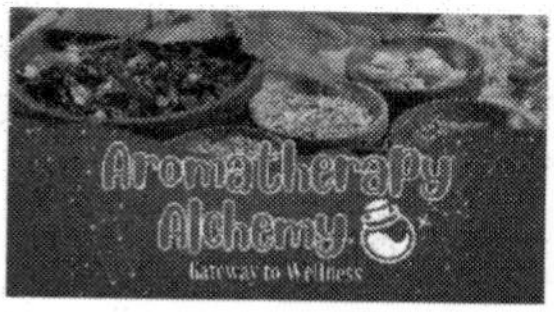

Aromatherapy Alchemy: Gateway to Wellness

Click to Sign Up

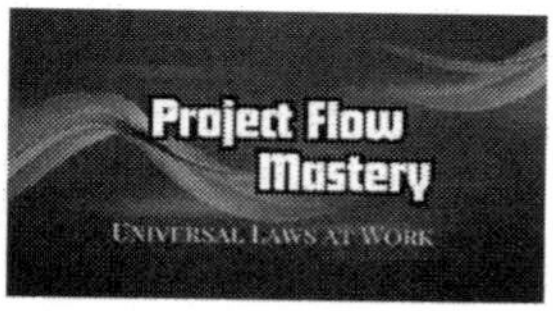

Project Flow Mastery: Universal Laws at Work

Click to Sign Up

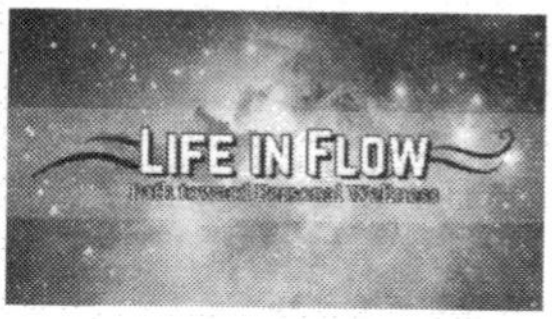

Life in Flow: Path Toward Personal Wellness

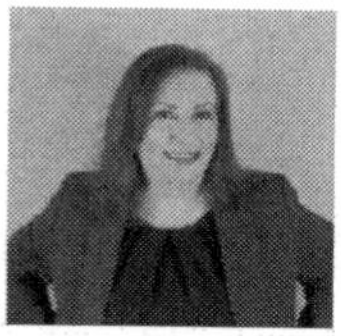

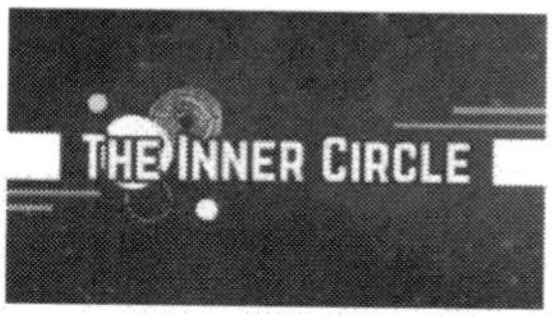

The Inner Circle

Free Groups:

https://www.facebook.com/groups/fundsfriendsfutures

https://www.facebook.com/groups/shifttimes

Also From TLM Publishing House

FICTION –

Sydney Brown Presents Series

https://www.amazon.com/dp/B0BSBT36HN

The Mall Cadet Series

https://www.amazon.com/gp/product/B0B66MDK3T

All In or Nothing Series

https://www.amazon.com/dp/B0B7FW9W8M

The 7 Wishes Series

https://www.amazon.com/dp/B0B62XJY59

The Deception Series

https://www.amazon.com/dp/B0B5RNQMF1

The Forbidden Love Series (18+)

https://www.amazon.com/dp/B0B5SX24SX

NONFICTION –

How to Start It Series

https://www.amazon.com/dp/B09Y2QHDPM

Aromatherapy Alchemy

https://www.amazon.com/dp/B0CJ5DD5C1